HOPE
for Cancer Patients
at All Stages of Illness

HOPE
for Cancer Patients at All Stages of Illness

Caring with more than just medicine

Radhakrishna Vemuri, M.D.

gatekeeper press™
Columbus, Ohio

Hope for Cancer Patients at All Stages of Illness
Caring with more than just medicine

Published by Gatekeeper Press
2167 Stringtown Rd, Suite 109
Columbus, OH 43123-2989
www.GatekeeperPress.com

Copyright © 2022 by Radhakrishna Vemuri

All rights reserved. Neither this book, nor any parts within it may be sold or reproduced in any form or by any electronic or mechanical means, including information storage and retrieval systems, without permission in writing from the author. The only exception is by a reviewer, who may quote short excerpts in a review.

The editorial work for this book is entirely the product of the author. Gatekeeper Press did not participate in and is not responsible for any aspect of this element.

Library of Congress Control Number: 2021940907

Paperback: 9781662914867
eISBN: 9781662914874

*Dedicated to my parents,
Ramakrishna (Nannagaru) and Sita (Amma),
with gratitude for their positive influence on me.
They taught me right from wrong,
the importance of having compassion
for my fellow human beings,
and how to remain free of self-destructive anger,
even when dealing with those who disagree.*

Contents

Author's Note ix
Foreword by the Author's Son xi
Preface xv

Chapter 1
The Importance of Compassionate Cancer Care 1

Chapter 2
Hope Is a Powerful Prescription 7

Chapter 3
Facing My Own Cancer Diagnosis 15

Chapter 4
Becoming A Doctor and Immigrating to the U.S. 23

Chapter 5
Hanging Out My Shingle 41

Chapter 6
Impactful Life Lessons 49

Chapter 7
A Balancing Act 59

Chapter 8
Challenges 69

Photo Section 81

Chapter 9
When the Truth is Not Enough 95

Chapter 10
The Three Categories of Patients 103

Chapter 11
Case Histories 113

Chapter 12
After Treatment 135

Chapter 13
Death Hits Close to Home 139

Chapter 14
The End of An Era 149

Afterword 155
About the Author 159
Acknowledgments 161
Works Cited 163

Author's Note

ALL LETTERS INCLUDED herein are from patients whom I treated unless expressly stated otherwise and are directly quoted from our correspondence. Out of respect to my patients and their right to privacy, most of the patients' names in this book have either been changed or omitted from patient cases, histories, and letters.

Foreword by the Author's Son

As a child, I thought of my father as primarily focused on his work as an oncologist and the Medical Director at the West Michigan Cancer Center. I knew that practicing medicine wasn't all he was about, of course. He regularly played tennis, badminton and golf. He spent hours on the phone with his large extended family, problem-solving with them or just catching up on their lives. He read my sister and me bedtime stories and made sure that we were very aware of it when our grades fell below the expected level.

So there was certainly more to him than work. And though oncology and the unavoidable sickness and death that a cancer doctor will always encounter can take an emotional toll on anyone, he clearly loved what he did and was very fulfilled by it. It always seemed that he managed to avoid burnout. When I was growing up I lost count of the number of times we'd run into former patients or their family members at the mall or a restaurant somewhere. They always talked about how much they loved my dad. It was striking, and I found it quite embarrassing as I became an adolescent, how much they would gush. When you sit down next to someone, surrounded by their loved ones, and tell them they have cancer, it is some of the worst news any of them can imagine. And still these people loved him and remembered him fondly. In some cases the patient had passed away but their family was still so warm and so glad to see him. He was great at holding people's hands, as my mom said.

I always assumed that my dad would keep working for as long as he could. It was clear that his professional life was important to him. When he started discussing retiring in a few years I expected him to push off the date. But he didn't, and as retirement got closer he started talking more and more about writing a book. It surprised me, as I had never known him to write; or even to read much other than medical journals. But what I had missed about his life and career was that he was always an educator. He was on the faculty of the Michigan State University Medical School and had won several educator of the year awards during his time there. He took pride in mentoring his interns and residents. He gave talks about the "Art of Medicine" to try to spread more of what he had learned throughout his career. From his perspective, the empathy that he showed his patients wasn't just his singular gift: it could be taught. And his equanimity and lack of burnout in his difficult field were things that other physicians could achieve as well.

A few years into retirement he was keeping busy playing tennis, golf, and working on his book. He was busy recording anecdotes, getting permission to use patients' stories and letters, and reading more than he had ever had time to while still practicing medicine. He was making progress, though it was slow. Then, during one summer visit to my parents' house, we all noticed a change in him. He was disoriented. He was forgetting things, and his balance seemed off. It was shocking and too steep and sudden a decline to be explained just by aging. We thought he might have had a stroke and speculated about other possibilities.

After some encouragement, he went into the hospital for tests. The diagnosis came back: cancer. One spot in his lung and more in his brain. The prognosis did not seem hopeful; something that he knew better than the rest of us. His book was certainly not at the front of my mind then, but it was uncertain whether he would finish it.

My dad underwent whole brain radiation due to the multiple metastases in his brain. He also received stereotactic radiation to a persistent spot in the right frontal lobe of his brain a year later. Both of these treatments were familiar to him from his time treating patients of his own. His oncologist also started him on Osimertinib, a targeted treatment that had not been available when he was practicing. These treatments helped significantly; the number of tumors decreased and the ones that remained shrank. His awareness and coordination improved as well. The followup tests and scans brought good news and one day on the phone he started talking to me about his book again. He said that with all the years he had spent understanding cancer and illness as a physician, administrator, educator and family member, this time as a patient would complete the picture. He is now taking his targeted treatment pill on a daily basis and plans to continue for as long as it helps him. With this treatment, he has been able to finally work on his book, collecting excerpts of writing from the past and combining them with patient letters and more recent thoughts.

And now he has actually finished that book. No matter what your experience with cancer, I hope that you are able to get something from it.

—Naveen Vemuri

Preface

I HAVE ALWAYS ENJOYED playing golf and tennis and I took some amount of pride in my abilities in both. My golf handicap was in the respectable seven to ten range and playing doubles tennis felt easy to me. I managed to win club championships in my respective divisions of both sports in 2015. Yet, just one year after that successful season, I found myself seeking further instruction in both as my talents seemed to have all but disappeared. I didn't think much of it at the time, not in a big picture sense. I just tried to address the problem as I saw it by signing up for lessons.

I did not even realize, at the time, that those lessons were not particularly beneficial. In spite of all the practice I was putting in, I continued to struggle with the games I loved and depended upon to maintain my life balance.

It was in 2017, while attending a family function that I first really noticed there might be something wrong with me. As someone who has always taken pride in my memory and thought process, I was suddenly aware that both were starting to show signs of waning. Perhaps through the power of denial, I continued to live my life without any major problems until June of 2018, when my wife and children began pointing out changes that they had noticed in regard to my physical and mental acuity. My attention span was notably shorter and my physical agility was not as sharp as it had been my entire life.

Eventually, I started acknowledging some of these changes for myself, such as occasional balance issues. I had no other worrisome symptoms such as headaches, however, and did not think much of the issue. I have always taken great pride in my skills as a clinician, which was reinforced by feedback received from colleagues and medical residents under my tutelage. Despite my belief that I was fine, I agreed to go see my primary care internist who then referred me to a neurologist. The specialist was thorough and scheduled an MRI (Magnetic Resonance Imaging) scan of my brain.

When given a chance to review the scans myself, I had no doubt what I was seeing. At least a dozen spots accompanied by considerable edema (swelling) were evident in my brain. I knew that this could mean only one thing; that cancer had metastasized from elsewhere in my body. Even filled with these spots, my brain was functional enough to realize what my next move had to be. The answer was the same whether I was the doctor or the patient.

I scheduled myself for a whole body CT (Computerized Tomography) scan to identify the source of the cancer. I prescribed Dexamethasone (Decadron) for myself to reduce the brain edema. My neurologist would have done the same but I could not entirely take off my "doctor hat" just yet. Even now, years into my treatment, I review every scan and regimen myself with a clinician's eye.

It is only in retrospect that I realize I was having symptoms two full years before my initial diagnosis. It was even earlier than that when I started writing this book, something I had wanted to do for decades. It was not until I was sick, however, that I really committed to finishing this project.

I was inspired to record the experiences I had as an oncologist because of my deeply held belief that hope is an essential and integral part of cancer care. In my thirty-five years in patient care, I was constantly reminded of the fact that the emotional and psychological aspects of cancer are every bit as impactful as the physical aspects of the disease. With this in mind, a well-rounded and compassionate approach to treatment is needed for all cancer patients regardless of their individual prognosis or life expectancy.

I was involved, either directly or indirectly, in the care of every patient I describe in this book. In these pages, appear some of the letters I received from patients, expressing their emotional reactions to their diagnoses, treatments, and sometimes, even their recoveries. I have also included some stories and letters from family members who have lost their loved ones under my care. Those whose personal correspondence I have included in this book were happy to share their experiences and emotions as an inspiration to others.

CHAPTER 1

The Importance of Compassionate Cancer Care

It is my firm assertion that the inspiration given by hope is the very centerpiece of compassionate cancer care. Hope is to the mind and emotions what surgery, chemotherapy, radiation therapy, and immunotherapy are to the bodies of cancer patients.

When a patient receives a cancer diagnosis, they experience many powerful emotions and are usually bombarded with a flood of conflicting thoughts. Overwhelmed with concerns and fears, their mind becomes chaotic. Some of their concerns are well-founded and some of their fears will never come to pass. It is human nature to fear the unknown and the fight against cancer is filled with unknowns.

In the following letter, a patient of mine expresses her fears over her diagnosis and describes the role that hope played in her emotional well-being:

> *That day when they were looking at my mammogram, fear really set in. Then I talked to my surgeon, who had talked to you. I had a team of people who were going to help me. A small glimmer of hope.*
>
> *When I started treatment with you after surgery, I asked you questions about some of my*

biggest fears. You answered them honestly. As difficult as some of it was to hear, I knew that you were committed to helping me.

It was so frustrating trying to hold my hubby together, hold my kids together, and my mom, sisters, brothers, etc. As much as people were around, I felt like I couldn't tell them my thoughts because I would scare them. But I knew that you had hope, so I had hope.

You were always optimistic, and I held onto that in a way I'm not sure you understand—the value of you telling me that this was going to be treated like a chronic disease. I could deal with that! Your decision to treat my cancer aggressively saved my life. I truly believe that. I am forever indebted to you, my angel on earth.

In my experience, cancer patients seem to fall into two groups. People in the first group focus on the doom-and-gloom aspects of their diagnoses and become depressed. And of course, depression often leads to inactivity and lack of engagement with life which can, in turn, affect health and treatment outcomes.

The second group says to themselves something like, *Alright, this situation is not good. But I am going to do the best I can, accept my predicament, and try to live a life that is as close to normal as possible.* All things being equal (e.g. stage of disease, standard of care, etc.) the second group of patients seem to fare better with their cancer and live longer. I, myself, am part of this group.

Giving hope to cancer patients goes well beyond the physical cure, treatment, or improvement of the disease's physical manifestations. We must also address the emotional toll taken by cancer. Any treatment protocol that fails to address every facet of the disease is incomplete. During my tenure as the founding medical director of the West Michigan Cancer Center (WMCC) from 1994 until my retirement in 2011, we had a well-organized support system set up for our patients.

The Importance of Compassionate Cancer Care

My nurse, Cindy, took care of all my patients. When one called WMCC, she was their first point of contact. Thanks to her gentle, soft-spoken manner, the patients loved her. She would always answer their questions herself if she could. When patients had more technical inquiries such as issues related to medication side effects, Cindy would pass them along to me. She definitely made my life simpler, in addition to the invaluable assistance she provided to patients and families. I was fortunate to have her by my side at WMCC until I retired. To this day, we stay in touch and I consider her a dear friend.

While I was the medical director of the West Michigan Cancer Center, Theresa "Terry" McKay was the CEO. She was responsible for approving and implementing many of the compassionate care services offered to our patients. She did a wonderful job and we got along very well. She made the West Michigan Cancer Center a beautiful, highly functional organization.

Terry recruited Barbara, the wife of a patient, to function as the head of volunteer services. Barbara was instrumental in lining up our support services. She also came up with an excellent idea; to have patients who had been treated at WMCC volunteer as coaches and mentors to new patients with similar diagnoses. They also offered comfort in the form of serving coffee and hot chocolate to patients and doctors. Volunteers play a major role in passing along the message of hope. This approach helps relieve new patients of some of the stress they experience. It also helps them find acceptance and better tolerance for chemotherapy.

The following is a letter from one of our volunteers. It highlights the importance of expressing gratitude to those who spend their time in the service of others:

> A few weeks ago, I came to my volunteer job at the Cancer Center feeling a little down and underappreciated. Then I encountered you, and you expressed your gratitude for the work that we volunteers do—whether it be greeting, coaching, pushing the coffee cart or whatever.

> *I have to tell you that your kind words made all the difference in the world to me! I perked up and faced the day with a revived spirit and joy. So, this note is to thank you for making such a difference in just a few words. You were so kind and thoughtful.*
>
> *Thank you again! Since you took the time to talk to me, I can only imagine how well you treat your patients.*

We also had financial counselors at the Center, personally selected and overseen by Terry. These counselors helped patients who could not afford expensive cancer treatments by reaching out to pharmaceutical companies and eliciting donations of free medications. They also coordinated with insurance companies on behalf of our patients, which anybody who has had medical care knows can be very helpful.

When our patients had exhausted all treatment options, a hospice team with dedicated nurses made a huge difference in maintaining their quality of life. The following is a letter sent to me by the surviving family of a patient of mine who passed away after receiving hospice care at the Center:

> *This is the most difficult card to write because we know you came to care for Junia very much. It was clearly seen in your wonderful way of dealing with her over the years. You gave her the hope she needed to carry on. She relied on your support and words of encouragement as well as your skill as a doctor.*
>
> *Even when you had to tell her that nothing more could be done, you did it gently so that she could absorb it and come to terms with it. She did fail very quickly. We are grateful you saw her promptly so hospice care could be given. The*

> family wants to thank you and your amazing staff for five years of giving and caring.
> You told Junia that the definition of hope may change over time. What never changed was your kindness to all of us and your loving care of Junia. May God bless you for all you have done for so many.

We used a hospice-like system even for those patients who were not in the end stages of the disease. We offered pain management, acupuncture, comfort, and music. We also offered exercise classes and yoga, both of which were very popular.

The following letter is from a volunteer at a hospice facility unaffiliated with WMCC, relating sentiments expressed to her by patients who enjoyed the hospice-type care at our facility:

> I have wanted to send you a note for quite some time. I have worked at a local hospice facility for over six years as a bereavement counselor. I have had the privilege of working with many bereaved individuals after the death of their loved ones.
> So many people have, over the years, talked so highly of you and the care you provided to them. They have shown me personal letters you have sent to them, and talked about the incredible sense of relief it has given them to know that you not only care about their physical needs but the emotional needs of them and their families.
> For this I am greatly thankful to you. Thank you for your kindness and love for the people you serve.

Individual and group counseling was made available to patients, as well. The group sessions were organized around commonality of cancer type. Knowing they were in a room with those facing the same issues brought patients great comfort and utilized the power of identification that has made groups like Alcoholic Anonymous so effective.

While it might be impossible to accurately quantify the effect of such holistic therapies on the cancer itself, there is no question that they support and enhance the overall wellness of the patient. I am living proof that they can both improve *quality* of life for the patient and extend *duration* of life. Dealing with my own cancer diagnosis as an oncologist has been its own adventure and has allowed me to truly practice what I preach.

Of course, I am far from the only cancer patient who has benefited greatly from a positive attitude and hopeful outlook. Scientific studies[1] [2] have proven the beneficial effect of a cancer patient's outlook and attitude on life expectancy and quality of life.

CHAPTER 2

Hope Is a Powerful Prescription

Once you choose hope, anything is possible.
—Christopher Reeve[3]

It is my fervent wish that as you read through this book; you, too, will find hope. It truly is a powerful prescription. When we feel hope, we must believe that our hope is well founded, perhaps due to a trust in science, a higher power, or even in ourselves.

Dr. Jerome Groopman, author of Anatomy of Hope, distinguishes true hope from "false hope," which he defines as the pervasive belief that everything will turn out fine.[4] We often hear the phrase, "Oh, everything will be okay." Doctors frequently use this phrase to console patients, even when the sentiment is empty and unfounded. True hope, on the other hand, is comprised of three elements—evidence, personal experience, and acceptance.

In his 1981 commentary entitled Hope, Howard Brody questions whether physicians truly have the power to take away a patient's hope. He concludes that while physicians do indeed possess the power to take away the hope of their patients, they do not have the authority to do so.[5]

One way that physicians inadvertently rob their patients of hope is by providing statistics and numbers about their odds of survival. A doctor could argue that they told the patient the truth, but the truth is not enough, not without context and explanations.

Physicians have the responsibility to provide all essential information to the patient. This can only be accomplished by a real conversation between doctor and patient that includes an explanation of the disease itself, including the science behind it and all treatment options. The physician must also talk to the patient about what they can expect with the recommended treatment and with alternate treatment options as applicable. It is important to include information about how this might impact the patient's quality of life and the lives of their loved ones and caretakers.

Adapting Hope to the Individual Patient

All cancer patients need hope but it is not a one-size-fits-all solution. As physicians, we need to adapt hope to each individual patient. I had a woman named Mary come to me for a second opinion after her first oncologist told her that she had a life expectancy of four months or less. She was a sixty three-year-old woman who had been diagnosed with metastatic pancreatic cancer. The prognosis given to Mary was, technically, accurate. While her original physician had told Mary the truth, he had failed to talk to her about all the essential elements of her diagnosis. He had not discussed with her how her cancer, its treatment, and consequently her life expectancy would impact her both physically and emotionally.

We can empower a patient by including them in all aspects of their own care and leaving in their hands the ultimate decision regarding how to proceed with treatment. Keeping the patient informed and involved in the decision-making process instills confidence and gives them hope.

When it comes to cancer patients, hope means different things to different people. Hope is not necessarily synonymous with a cure or even with cancer survival, as one might think. Its meaning will vary from patient to patient and can even change as the patient moves through the stages of their illness.

Over the course of my long career in oncology, I learned how to define hope at every stage of cancer without distorting reality or deviating from the truth in communication with patients. For those with an early diagnosis who are on a protocol of proven useful treatment, the definition of hope is a cure.

For patients with cancers which are treatable but not curable, the definition of hope is to increase the *quantity* of life and to improve the *quality* of life. This brand of hope is possible thanks to ever-improving treatments in the field of cancer which allow the disease to become chronic without being fatal, the way many people live with diabetes, arthritis, or asthma. These patients may live long enough that their eventual cause of death is unrelated to their initial cancer diagnosis. I once had a fifty eight-year-old patient who came to me suffering from renal cancer with lung metastasis. Once his cancerous kidney was removed, his health improved and he lived a full life until he died of an unconnected heart attack in his seventies.

Another patient who fell into this category was Linda, a forty two-year-old woman who came to me in April of 2005 with stage IV breast cancer. Her cancer had metastasized to her lymph nodes, bones, and liver. I explained to her that although there was no cure for her cancer, hope was not lost. She underwent chemotherapy treatment with a hopeful outlook, despite being quite anxious when I first met her. After chemotherapy, she continued to do well. In fact, in June of 2020, I was delighted to receive an email from her, letting me know that she is still alive and maintaining an excellent quality of life. Linda was one of my inspirations for writing this book.

For those patients who reach a stage where further treatments would cause more harm than benefit, the definition of hope is comfort, both physical and emotional. I arrived at this conclusion through many years of caring for patients with widely advanced malignancy that was obvious at presentation or whose cancers progressed despite proven treatments.

In talking with these patients, I discovered that the majority were aware of their grim prognoses. Yet, they were more afraid of pain and suffering than they were of dying. That is how I came to the conclusion that for these patients, hope is comfort.

In her book <u>On Death and Dying</u>, Elizabeth Kubler-Ross writes about the five stages of grief experienced by patients with a terminal diagnosis. These include denial and isolation, anger, bargaining, depression, and acceptance.[6] Not all patients go through each stage, of course, and the stages do not always occur in that order. However, I observed that patients do go through such a process as they try to gain a better understanding of their medical condition and its implications.

When physicians fail to give patients a well-rounded understanding of their condition, it can lead to anxiety. Simply hearing that a treatment is available can make a significant difference in a patient's outlook.

Once a patient has a good understanding of what is going on with their cancer, they tend to become much more confident and hopeful. This is why connecting patients with others who have the same diagnosis can be very reassuring. They get to talk to someone who has gone through the same things that they have from discovery through treatment.

Giving patients options can be very reassuring to them. For example, if a patient is afraid of the side effects of chemotherapy, I might discuss with them whether we can modify the treatment without jeopardizing the outcome. A great example of this is when we offer breast cancer patients anti-hormone pills which allow them to receive treatment at home. They still need to come in to see the physician for monitoring but most days they can remain in a familiar and comfortable environment. A similar example can be found in the treatment of men with prostate cancer. Just like the way that breast cancer in women is often fed by estrogen and/or progesterone, prostate cancer is fed by testosterone. We can give these men anti-testosterone injections to starve the cancer or put it in abeyance.

Offering to modify treatments for patients in such a way that they are better able to cope gives them hope which, as we know, is central to the emotional well-being of patients. Hope can improve the prognosis of a patient by improving their outlook and their overall sense of well-being. When patients are hopeful, their state of mind can have a notable positive impact on their therapeutic treatment.

Never Give Up

When a patient is hopeful and optimistic, and keeps a positive attitude, it fortifies them and gives them the strength needed to keep fighting their cancer battle. I recently received a letter from a former patient of mine named Myrna. She came to me with breast cancer after seeing a previous oncologist. Her story beautifully illustrates the importance of maintaining a positive attitude.

> I first learned that I had breast cancer when I had a mammogram in October of 1993. I was horrified and disbelieving because I had never felt fitter than I did right then. When my family and friends learned of my diagnosis, they started telling me about herbs, diets and many other ways to fight the cancer.
>
> One of these alternative "cures" was an electrical box. It was presented to me by a loved one who told me that standing on the box and receiving multiple shocks would rid me of cancer. The box did not cure me of cancer but it did cure me of listening to any more goofy ideas. From then on, I kept my focus on what the doctors told me to do.
>
> I, like everyone else, despised cancer and decided that if it attacked me, I was going to attack it in return. So, I told my husband that surgery was likely to be a better way to rid myself of cancer. He agreed.
>
> A surgical biopsy done a couple of weeks later revealed that cancer was in eight of the twenty-six lymph nodes that were removed. I was shocked and thought it was a bad sign. Then I said to myself, Well, maybe they got it all.
>
> I went for my first appointment with an oncologist. He was very negative during the

entire appointment. Afterward, I went to the front desk and requested another oncologist. Then I remembered my neighbor Bobby who worked at Borgess Hospital for twenty years. He told me about a doctor who he described as "very good." That doctor turned out to be you.

Asking you to be my doctor was one of the best decisions of my life and for my life. Thank you, my friend, for being the wonderful doctor that you are in every way possible.

I had surgery, went through a clinical study, and then took Tamoxifen which you prescribed to me. I remember you telling me at the time, "It only works for five years."

Sure enough, in the eleventh year, the cancer came back in my lymph nodes. So, I underwent radiation. I never had any dread of appointments or scans because you always had such a positive attitude.

You entered the room at each appointment saying, "I have nothing bad to say." We talked about my photography, my husband's sports, and your tennis and golf.

One morning, I had a scare when I went into the bathroom and spit up blood. My doctor recommended an immediate scan but you disagreed. You told me that every now and then a tiny blood vessel can break. You said, "If it continues, we will look into it." What a great tool it is, knowing I don't have to worry about every little thing.

Early in 1994, I finished up my third and final chemotherapy. Long ago I learned two rules:

Rule number 1: Never, ever give up.
Rule number 2: Never forget rule number 1.

This letter arrived twenty-eight years after Myrna's initial diagnosis. She had multiple nodes that returned and received further chemotherapy treatment. Due to positive hormone receptors, she also received anti-estrogen treatment.

Whenever I see a patient with metastatic cancer, I hesitate to use the word "cured." There are, of course, always those who are outliers and exceptions. What I can say with certainty is that Myrna is currently eighty-eight years old and free of breast cancer. While she is naturally experiencing some age-related slowing and hearing problems, Myrna is living a normal life, and even won an award recently for her photography!

CHAPTER 3

Facing My Own Cancer Diagnosis

The Shocking News

I HAD NO IDEA, when I started thinking about writing this book, that I would become a living example of my message of hope. It happened in July of 2018 when I received an unexpected diagnosis of lung cancer which had metastasized to my brain. I was given a life expectancy at that time of only six to eight months.

I have no words to describe how shocked I was when the doctor first gave me that news. My heart stopped for a moment. I asked myself, *Can this be real?*

Following My Own Prescription

Despite my dire prognosis, here I am nearly four years later, still among the living. I continue to feel great and maintain a good quality of life on target-based treatment. I can even participate in my favorite physical activities of golf and tennis. It was my cancer diagnosis that hastened the writing of this book, which I had been putting off for many years. Having already exceeded my own life expectancy many times over, I was even more inspired to write about hope now that I had experience from the other side of the exam table.

Of course, I could not help but look at my own test results with a physician's eye. On countless occasions during my tenure as an oncologist, I had looked at similar scans. There was no doubt in my mind what the images meant—cancer. It was both no different and miles away from the plethora of scans I had seen before.

When I first went to see a doctor, I had no pulmonary symptoms. Lung cancer was the last thing on my mind. The issues that sent me to get this scan were neurological in nature; balance and memory issues, mostly. As I looked at the evidence however, it was clear, I realized that I had metastatic cancer in my brain and it had to have originated somewhere.

I quickly adjusted from reacting like a patient to seeing things as an oncologist. This allowed me to regain my calm and composure. I knew that I was no different than the myriad patients I had seen during my career and I asked myself, *If these scans belonged to a patient of mine, what would I do next to treat them?* The answer came to me fairly readily. I knew that I had to do what I had done countless times during my years of practicing oncology. I had to properly diagnose the disease.

First, I called in a prescription to the local pharmacy for dexamethasone; a long-acting corticosteroid with anti-inflammatory properties which is four to five times more effective than the more common steroid, prednisone. I prescribed this to myself in order to reduce the swelling in my brain and to prevent a possibly fatal brain herniation as well as to provide immediate symptom relief.

Secondly, I scheduled an appointment for a full-body computerized tomography (CT) scan to take place the following day. I knew the scan would identify the original source of the cancer which had metastasized to my brain. On July 18th, 2018, I underwent the scan. The results showed a mass in my left lung that measured 3.2 by 2.9 centimeters, or about the size of a half dollar. This was presumably the source of my brain metastases.

One week later, on July 25th, 2018, I underwent a CT-guided needle biopsy of the lung mass. Ensuing tests confirmed the diagnosis of adenocarcinoma. As I went through each test and discussed the results with my oncologist, my mind was in constant motion between thinking like a patient and thinking like a doctor.

The following is an excerpt from an article written by Jo Cavallo after interviewing me about my cancer diagnosis for TAP: The Patient's Corner:

"The diagnosis came as a surprise because except for some minor neurologic symptoms, including subtle changes in my memory and balance which I thought might be the result of a transient ischemic attack, I felt fine. However, the symptoms were bothersome enough for me to seek medical attention from a neurologist.

"Based on the neurologic exam, the doctor ordered a brain Magnetic Resonance Imaging (MRI), which detected multiple lesions in my brain, including two masses more than 4 cm in my right frontal-parietal and temporal lobes with surrounding edema. Having seen hundreds of similar images from scans of patients I've treated over the years, I immediately knew the significance of these lesions, but I had no emotional reaction."[7]

Note: The entire article can be found on The ASCO Post's website.

The Gift of Acceptance

Interestingly, I did not have any real emotional reaction to the findings. My mind was blank at the time of the diagnosis confirmation and it remained that way throughout the rest of the day. I can only attribute this deviation from the way most people react to such a terrible diagnosis to one very simple thing: a habitual attitude of acceptance.

The seeds of this immediate acceptance can be traced all the way back to my teen years. That is when my father (whom I called Nannagaru, a term of paternal respect in our language) told me, "Son, unexpected events occur which you have no control over. The only control you have in such situations is how you react. So, it's your mind that you should train."

My emotional equilibrium has also been heavily influenced by the many lessons I have learned from the *Bhagavad Gita*. The *Gita* (as it is often colloquially known) is an ancient holy text, a 700-verse Hindu scripture dating back to the second century BCE. It is part of the epic Mahabharata, the longest poem ever written. The *Gita* is, in broad strokes, a conversation between the hero, Pandava Prince Arjuna, and his mentor, Krishna, an avatar of the god Vishnu. The spiritual teachings of the *Gita* had a significant influence on me. There are three major lessons which can apply to all of our lives:

> **Dharma**. This is a sacred duty that we must fulfill during our lifetime. Sacred duty refers to the moral order that sustains the society and the individual. We can all use this idea to help us cope with our responsibilities in life and see them as our duties rather than as burdens.
>
> **Disciplined Action**. In difficult times we stop, paralyzed with fear and doubt. The lesson here is to never stop turning the wheels set in motion. When we do, we waste our lives and bring our growth to a standstill.
>
> **Self-knowledge**. There is one unchanging thing and that is self—our true essence. The answers do not lie in the external world. They lie within us. We must part the clouds of ignorance with self-knowledge. It is best to focus on the attempt and not the result.[8]

Beating the Odds

I was fortunate to see a friendly, knowledgeable radiation specialist who recommended whole-brain radiation, my treatment of choice. I underwent two weeks of radiation which was administered in ten treatment fractions and completed on August 10th, 2018.

My next stop was the office of a medical oncologist with expertise in lung cancer. Since my retirement seven years before, there had been significant advances in lung cancer treatment, with the identification of multiple targets in the cancer cells. The oncologist ordered a lung biopsy and the specimen was sent to the lab in order to identify targets that could influence the type of treatment which would be most beneficial to me. My oncologist was excited to report that my cancer was positive for epidermal growth factor receptor (EGFR), a protein found on the surface of cells. Mutations of this protein can lead to growth and spread of cancer cells. The reason that this was a fortunate result is that there are currently four agents targeting EGFR which are FDA approved and available for treating lung cancer. Before initiating systemic treatment for my lung cancer, the doctor ordered a baseline CT scan, which was performed on August 21st.

When the results of the CT scan came back, I got a pleasant surprise. The scan showed that the mass in my lung had spontaneously been reduced by 30%, without any treatment at all to address my lung cancer! In July of 2018, on the day of my diagnosis, the tumor had been the size of a half dollar. Now, barely a month later, it had shrunk to 2.1 x 2.4 cm, closer to the size of a quarter. The exact mechanism of this spontaneous reduction is not known. This phenomenon only confirmed for me that there is much we don't know about cancer and the body's response to it.

I said to myself, *Hopefully this is a prelude to the future behavior of my cancer!*

My oncologist is treating me with Osimertinib, a third-generation EGFR tyrosine kinase inhibitor. To date, this medication is keeping the cancer stable and I feel almost as good as I did five years ago. My brain continues to be stable with persistent but smaller lesions, and for the most part, I remain free of symptoms. I still periodically undergo follow-up positron emission tomography (PET) / CT scans and MRIs to make sure that everything remains under control.

At the time of my diagnosis, I was aware that my statistical life expectancy was only six to eight months. Yet, I have clearly proven that to be an inaccurate estimation. There are a few possible explanations for such an outcome.

First of all, similar cancers do not necessarily share a common path. One must consider factors such as variations in immune response, differences in biology in the cell lines, and variations in patient attitude and behavior.

In my particular case, I have habitually and consistently lived my life with a positive outlook. There are undoubtedly other factors in play, as well; factors which are impossible to identify or quantify with any specificity or accuracy.

Despite my diagnosis, I continue to live a full life and keep busy. I give second opinions to members of my community who have cancer and blood disorders. I feel privileged to be able to share my expertise with others, an activity which has the side benefit of keeping my brain sharp and my knowledge up-to-date. I also play golf and tennis on a regular basis, which helps keep my body fit. I am an example of living a hopeful life even when a cure is not a realistic option. Many people want to know how I retain such a hopeful outlook.

Instead of dwelling on my cancer diagnosis, I do my best to maintain normalcy in my daily routine. By physically keeping routine and structure in my life, my outlook automatically improves. With my brain engaged in one thing or the other, it does not give me much time to dwell on my diagnosis and any potentially serious consequences. This is not to say that I live in a constant state of denial. I understand my situation better than many others who share it, I simply choose not to let it control my life.

I believe that this approach to living as I am embraces the spirit of my message of hope at all states of cancer treatment and in other serious situations as well. Keeping the brain active and trying to maintain as much of a normal routine as possible is the key. Exercise is an essential part of my normal routine. Interestingly, exercise is more effective than any medicine when it comes to addressing cancer-related fatigue. It is the antidote to both the physical and emotional aspects of cancer, and the secret to an enhanced sense of well-being.

The Role of Radon Gas in Lung Cancer

After my diagnosis, I pondered the question of what might have caused my lung cancer as I am a lifelong nonsmoker without known risk factors.

I began looking into my possible radon exposure, knowing that it is the number-one cause of lung cancer in nonsmokers, according to EPA estimates. In fact, overall, radon is the second leading cause of lung cancer. It is responsible for about 21,000 lung cancer deaths every year, about 2,900 of which occur in nonsmokers. On January 13, 2005, Dr. Richard H. Carmona, the U.S. Surgeon General, issued a national health advisory on radon.[9]

Radon is a colorless, odorless radioactive gas. It forms naturally from the decay of the radioactive element uranium, found in soil and rocks worldwide in varying amounts. Radon gas escapes into the air as well as underground and surface water. The EPA has established a radon level of 4 pCi/L as a benchmark at which action needs to be taken to reduce the chances of developing lung cancer. The unit of pCi/L, or picocuries per liter, is a measure of how much radioactive decay is taking place in a given volume of air.

The national average indoor radon level is 1.3 pCi/L. The average indoor radon levels in the county where I live, as determined by radon test results from Air Chek, Inc. is 2.5 pCi/L. Twenty-eight percent of homes in the community have levels of 4 pCi/L.[10]

When a person is exposed to radon, the radioactive particles further decay into various nuclides. Some of these are harmless while others can be a significant source of both alpha (α) and beta (β) radiation. When alpha particles damage a cell to make it cancerous, the onset of lung cancer takes a minimum of five years, but most often much longer. I am aware of two other nonsmoking members of my community with non-small-cell adenocarcinoma of the lung, the most common lung cancer among non-smokers.

CHAPTER 4

Becoming A Doctor and Immigrating to the U.S.

*The good physician treats the disease;
the great physician treats the patient who has the disease.*
—Sir William Osler[11]

My Origin Story

On August 22ND, 1948, I was delivered at home by a midwife in my mother's hometown of Masulipatnam, located 150 miles from the large South Indian city of Hyderabad. We moved to Hyderabad when I was a baby and I consider it to be my hometown, although with over six million residents in the city itself, perhaps "town" is a bit of an understatement.

While I am proud to say that I became a United States citizen in 1980, I regret that I had to renounce my native Indian citizenship to do so. Consequently, whenever I want to visit the country of my birth, I have to apply for a visa like any other foreign tourist. As my children and grandchildren are all native-born Americans, however, this country is now my true home.

When I was three years old, I fell ill with smallpox, a disease which has since been globally eradicated, and was admitted to the hospital with a high fever along with my elder sister. Thankfully, after only a few days, we both fully recovered and were able to return home. Our parents learned a lesson from the scare and had all of our younger siblings vaccinated. Our family was very fortunate as many people died of the disease in India at that time.

Although I recovered completely from smallpox, it left me with a scarred face. Consequently, for most of my childhood, I found myself an object of ridicule due to my pock marks. This caused me considerable distress and took a major toll on my confidence and self-esteem. Although I have since been able to overcome the extreme self-consciousness that came from my smallpox scars, I am very happy to know that since 1980, not a single child has had to suffer the same trauma I endured in childhood.

I am the second eldest of my parents' eight children and the eldest male. We are evenly split among gender lines, giving me three each; younger brothers and sisters. All eight of us have always been very close, even today with half of us on each side of the globe. Our fondness for each other and inside jokes persist. They still tease me about assigning them homework as children and I still maintain that it was good for them! All of us are college-educated and half of us hold advanced degrees.

The sibling closest in age to me is Sudhakar, only sixteen months my junior. We were best friends throughout our childhood and, as typical boys, we were mischievous together in mostly harmless ways; stealing fruit from neighbors' fruit trees and getting into fights with other kids. One of our favorite misbehaviors was to sneak into movie theaters during the intermission. What was playing never mattered too much, we were more interested in the thrill of the caper than the film itself. In 2013, Sudhakar was diagnosed with Chronic Lymphocytic Leukemia (CLL) which I helped him manage without medical treatment for eight years until he passed away of COVID in May of 2021. CLL can be managed in some patients without intervention because the treatment available, which reduces white blood cell count, does not alter the natural course of the disease when given at early stages and is ultimately not recommended as it may cause side effects without any benefit.

As a teacher, my father took an intense interest in my education. He knew the importance of English as the world's business language and saw the mastery of it as an important step toward a successful future. Toward this goal, he sent me to a private school where all of the courses were taught in English and the teachers were American. It may sound odd that I attended a Methodist school but it was well worth it for the opportunity to learn in English. Although Nannagaru was a kind and, in many ways, progressive man, he was also a disciplinarian with unbendable rules about completing our homework on the same day it was assigned; there was no procrastination in our house! My father's lessons served me well and I graduated from Methodist Boys High School at the tender age of fifteen.

While our father maintained control over our formal education, it was our mother who was in charge of our emotional development. Amma, as we called her, often used proverbs to teach us all important lessons. In addition to teaching us in theory, she always led by example. I never saw her get angry or raise her voice to discipline any of her eight often mischievous children. Not once did I ever hear her utter a negative word or be critical of another person. She has always been my role model for generosity and tact.

Although my parents had more children than money, they were still able to provide us with many happy memories. One highlight of my childhood was our annual visit to my father's birthplace in the Krishna District of Andhra Pradesh. There were large mango fields in my father's village, and we children always had a wonderful time plucking ripe mangoes straight from the tree. I have fond memories of these trips and I can still taste the mangoes; the king of Indian fruit. My favorite was the "juice" variety of mango. By making a small hole and massaging the fruit in a certain way, we could squeeze copious amounts of juice directly into our mouths.

Like many people's early years, mine were something of a mixed bag. One incident from my childhood that I will never forget occurred when I was only seven years old. Along with two other boys, I played truant from school and spent the afternoon at a playground. While enjoying my freedom, I fell off a swing and injured my foot. At the time, I did not realize that anything was wrong but at two o'clock in the morning, I awoke in excruciating pain. I needed help but was too afraid to tell Nannagaru about my disobedience. Instead, I made up a story about a scorpion biting me while I was walking through the backyard on my way to the bathroom, which was outside at that time.

My father took his flashlight out into the backyard where he scoured the ground for at least half an hour in search of a nonexistent scorpion. Meanwhile, I was crying from the pain in my foot. My father only ceased his quest in order to carry me to the home of a doctor friend who lived nearby.

By the time I saw the doctor, both my foot and ankle had swollen profusely and were tender to the touch. The doctor sent me home with an ointment and some pain medication. Although we had an open and honest relationship, I never did tell my father what had really happened to cause my injury.

Playing Doctor

Another enjoyable part of my childhood involved playing make-believe with my friends. Sometimes we made up little plays. Sometimes, an older friend who acted as our leader would suggest an idea that would spark our imaginations. Our only audience was each other, but that did not take away from our fun. I had a large group of friends, so we never lacked for a crowd of spectators. We had never heard of improvisation games but we played one where we had to come up with silly answers to serious questions.

"Where are the gold mines in India?" My friend asked.

"Around my mother's neck!" I replied. It always seemed to me that she had plenty of jewelry. When we did skits and plays, our roles would vary. Sometimes, I wore a toy stethoscope and pretended to be a doctor. My advice to the patient, usually some younger playmate, was generally along the lines of, "Eat well and be strong!"

I still give out the same advice, although I tend to include more specifics today. My idea of good diet advice almost always included three foods in particular: peanuts, milk, and tomatoes. I was protein-conscious long before it was a diet trend and loved peanuts for that reason. Milk was delivered in glass bottles and kept very cold in the refrigerator. I always thought a chilled glass of milk was the most delicious thing that could pass my lips. The tomatoes did not fill a specific nutritional need as far as I knew but they were plump, red, juicy, and delicious.

Although we were a strictly vegetarian family, not all Hindus are, many eat certain types of meat but almost never beef. Cows are considered a sacred symbol of life to be revered and protected. This taboo does not extend to dairy products, however, which are a staple of many Hindu diets.

Despite my interest in nutrition, I do not recall any great longing to become a doctor when I was a child. I doubt that playing pretend like that had any real influence on my future profession. I think that I was too young to have been really making plans regarding a career path. I admit though that I did enjoy the feeling of authority I got by doling out basic health advice to my "patients."

Why I Became A Doctor

So, if it was not my childish games that ignited my interest in medicine, there must have been something else. The question of why I chose to become a doctor is not really the right one to ask; it was not my choice at all. My father made the decision on my behalf for what was both the most common reason mixed with a rather surprising and amusing one. Whatever his motivation though, I am glad he made the decision that he did. I will always be indebted to him for providing me with such a well-suited career path.

I learned the real reason that my father wanted his firstborn son to become a doctor when I received my acceptance letter from The Institute of Medical Sciences at Osmania Medical College in Hyderabad, India. It was May of 1964, still several months shy of my sixteenth birthday.

After I received the letter, my father explained why he was so motivated to get me into medical school. He had always wanted to be a doctor himself. Living one's dreams through children is, of course, an extremely common goal. However, it was not any failure or lack of ability that had kept my father from his dream vocation but rather the beliefs of his conservative parents. In fact, he was offered a seat at a prestigious medical college in Madras State in 1935, during the British rule of India. Unfortunately, my grandparents forbade their son from becoming a doctor. Their reasoning for this decision was simple although when looking at it with the wisdom of time past, it seems almost ludicrous today: rectal exams. They did not know everything a physician would have to do but they were undeniably aware of at least one unpleasant duty which was performed by doctors. That reason alone was enough for them to make sure my father never realized his dream.

How was the mere possibility of one single duty adequate to change the course of a young man's life forever? It boils down to India's rigid caste system which was, at that time, much more strict in practice than it is today. There are four castes (classes) defined in Hindu scriptures: Brahmins, priests and scholars; Kshatriyas, warriors and leaders; Vaishyas, merchants and farmers; and Shudras, laborers. There is some disagreement over what caste doctors (and other modern professions) should appropriately come from, one of many reasons the system is outdated today.

As Brahmans, my traditional grandparents deemed the work of a doctor to be unsuitable for my father, not because of the years of study involved, of course, but because of the impurity associated with rectal exams and likely other tasks they knew nothing about. It was an unclean thing and should not be asked of a member of the priestly caste. Consequently, my father became a school teacher and never even suggested that he resented his parents for forcing him down that path. That did not mean he would do the same to his children, of course.

I am sure that my father had the idea to nurture me, his eldest son, to become a doctor from the time of my birth. There is no doubt that he got vicarious pleasure from doing so, raising me to fulfill the dream that was denied to him. Nannagaru was also a progressive man. In 1970s India, he insisted on all of his daughters getting a college education and property of their own, never wanting them to have to rely solely on their husbands.

I do not recall that I personally had much of a reaction upon reading my acceptance letter to medical school but I clearly remember to this day the look of pride on my father's face while reading that letter. He had tears of pure happiness in his eyes. He made sure that I knew what I had accomplished; medical school admission was highly competitive. He told me that they received over eight thousand applications for only a hundred and fifty seats. I later realized that this was his way of ensuring that I studied hard and did not take the opportunity for granted.

One month before the commencement of my medical education, my father imparted to me some wisdom that set the tone for my entire medical career. To this day, I remember his exact words:

"Son," he said, "you will be entering into a noble profession. You need to treat every patient with utmost respect and compassion, and give them hope whenever possible, without deviating from the truth. Treat them the way you would like to be treated. Imagine yourself in their shoes to understand what they are going through."

My father's message helped me a great deal, not only during my thirty-five years as a practicing oncologist caring for patients who were sick and dying, but also in my life in general. He was the first to instill in me my belief in the all important nature of hope.

The Path to Medical School

In America these days, kids are often asked what they want to be when they grow up and whether they answer "princess" or "postal worker," they learn to think along those lines quite young, being told that they can be anything they want. In India when I was growing up, there were many fewer options than there are today, even setting aside the still crumbling barriers based on caste. The field of technology is booming in India today and even has many subcategories, but was still part of an unimaginable future when I was a child, before globalization had yet to really take hold.

At that time, those who wanted to earn a good living and garner respect became engineers or doctors. Other well-regarded vocations could be found at a bank or as a college professor. Four of my siblings worked in banks for many years. The limited options available to me prevented me from imagining as a child what I wanted to be when I grew up. Additionally, my father began to groom me to become a doctor when I was somewhere between the ages of ten and twelve. So, I never really questioned my future profession.

Doctors did not necessarily get a separate undergraduate education in India at that time. A student who had completed grade twelve could apply to medical school during the year in which they turned sixteen. Contingent upon good grades and test scores, of course.

The application and admissions period generally occurred in June. In 1963, I was fifteen years old and had just completed the twelfth grade. I would not turn sixteen until August of 1964. Even skipping what we think of in America as "college," that is pretty young to enter medical school. I do know of a few other young men who were admitted at my age.

Independently of my medical school application, I had received a full scholarship to attend college for a Bachelor of Science degree, which might have led me out of the medical field, or at least out of patient care, My father's determination to have his first son become a physician took priority, however, and I turned down the college admission and associated scholarship. Nannagaru felt that the extra year I had would be better spent improving my already excellent grades.

"Next year when you are sixteen," he explained, "there might be more competition. Instead of going to college now, why don't you use this next year to repeat the twelfth grade? That way, you can make your scores even higher."

My scores were already quite high but given the amount of competition for medical school I was likely to face when I came of age the following year, my father insisted that I needed the highest scores I could get.

It was not as easy as that, however. Repeating the twelfth grade required special permission from the Hyderabad Board of Education. It was unheard of for a student to repeat a grade without having failed it the first time through. While I have no data to corroborate this, I suspect that I may have been the first student with such high scores to ever make that sort of request to any Board of Education in India.

My father approached the Board of Education on my behalf. Before asking them whether I could repeat twelfth grade, he attempted a different tactic, which would have allowed me to apply to medical school that year. He tried to tell them that I was actually born in 1947 rather than 1948, as my birth certificate stated, making me sixteen years of age that August. If they had been willing to change my date of birth in my school records, I would have had a head start toward our goal.

The Board of Education rejected the idea, saying a more professional version of, "Nice try, but nothing doing!"

With his original plan rejected, my father then asked for permission to have me repeat grade twelve. He explained his desire to have me enter medical school and that going without schooling for the intervening year might leave me at a disadvantage. This request, the Board of Education approved.

Anatomy Lessons

In my second year of medical school, I was put on a team of four and assigned the task of dissecting a human body. We were paired up and given a dissection manual. Two of us were to dissect the legs, and the other two the arms. Our teacher told us, "If you'll just follow the manual, you will learn all about human anatomy." Instead of being given a replica body, we were given a real human cadaver to dissect. The cadaver had been preserved with formaldehyde, and the chemical smell was overwhelming. It was hardly surprising when one of our group dropped out because he could not take the smell. While the offensive odor bothered me terribly as well, I was able to work through it until I grew accustomed.

During the dissection process, we learned about the ligaments, muscles, nerves, blood vessels, and so on. Each day, the diener would place the cadaver on the table for dissection. Our cadaver was a female whom we named Cleopatra. Our supervisor got a chuckle out of that.

Dissecting a real human body rather than man made replicas was extremely educational. The first lesson I learned from that experience was that you cannot really get the true feeling of dissection when cutting into a replica. Incisions just are not the same. For anyone studying to become a surgeon, this would be even more important. As an oncologist, my career included less in the way of hands-on refreshers, but I found that my knowledge of human anatomy remained strong well into the later years of my practice. The second major lesson I learned while dissecting had more to do with human nature than the human body.

The following year, we were given a nerve-conduction assignment. The assignment involved dissecting a frog's calf muscle which was attached to the nerve. We connected it to an electrode which stimulated the muscle. It registered like an EKG although, of course, a calf muscle is a bit different than the heart. During the exam, I inadvertently cut through the nerve. Once that was severed, the muscle no longer functioned. The professor responded to my mistake with harsh criticism.

Not long afterward, a female student made the exact same mistake. The professor's reaction was to kindly place his hand on her shoulder and say, "Don't worry, these things happen."

I could hardly believe what I was hearing. We had made the same mistake and were of nearly equal standing, my class rank was only one ahead of hers. I thought to myself, *I can't believe this guy is being so critical of me and so nice to this girl!* I realized then that everybody has their own biases and ways of looking at the world. I felt determined that while I would always treat people equally well, sometimes reactions and approaches need to be tailored to individuals.

Final Exams

Medical school in India was a six-year program. We followed the British system, which involved passing exams related to both the theory and practice of medicine. These exams covered all clinical subjects and were given at the end of our final year, prior to graduation. By that time, I had already decided that after graduation, I would pursue a residency in internal medicine at the prestigious All India Institute of Medical Sciences in New Delhi.

Given that I have been in America for half a century now, it is clear that I was destined for a very different future than the one I had planned at that time. I do not regret for a moment that my original plans fell through. The life I went on to live was very fulfilling. And while I will never know what my life might have looked like had I stayed in India, I am content with the life I have today.

It was something that occurred during one of my practical exams that changed the course of my future as a doctor. I was assigned a sixteen-year-old male patient with a congenital disorder that predisposed him to frequent lung infections requiring hospitalization. On several occasions during my rotations through the internal medicine wards, I had seen this exact same patient. So, I was already familiar with his diagnosis and knew all about his history of lung infections.

When I was quizzed on this patient's condition by my British-trained professor, I was able to say with confidence what ailed him because I had become so familiar with his particular condition. This confidence came as a shock to the professor who clearly did not expect me, as a mere student, to be able to properly diagnose the patient. I was very cautious in the way I presented my knowledge of the patient's condition, not even making a formal diagnosis. Nevertheless, due to the examiner's bias, he jumped to the conclusion that the only way I could have known so much about the patient was if I had received a tip of some kind. Without any real evidence he was convinced that I had cheated.

I had initially felt encouraged by my wealth of knowledge concerning that patient's condition. Sadly, my triumph was short-lived. When accused of cheating, I told the truth, that my familiarity with the young patient was due to his multiple admissions during my internal medicine rotations. This perfectly reasonable explanation fell on deaf ears. Despite my best efforts, I could not get the professor to believe the truth; that I had not received help from any internal staff. The knowledge was my own and I had not cheated.

Despite the accusation of dishonesty, I received a passing grade in internal medicine. I was still able to graduate with top honors thanks to the gold medal awards I won in surgery and ob-gyn. The examining professor's accusations and refusal to listen discouraged me however. I felt that his preconceived notions about me overshadowed my obvious capabilities. I realized that this was not the sort of environment in which I wished to continue my education and began considering alternatives to the All India Institute.

That incident changed not only my future plans for residency in India, but the entire rest of my life. I had not ever intended to leave India and come to the United States to practice medicine but I suddenly found myself in a position where it seemed like my best option. I am certainly glad that I chose to emigrate. I have had incredible professional and personal satisfaction being a physician, particularly an oncologist. I have made friends here whom I could never do without and, of course, had I not made the decision I did, I would never have met my American wife, Karen, who has added unquantifiable value to my life in many ways.

Leaving India

Having determined to try my luck outside of India, I decided to join some of my classmates in taking the exam offered by the Educational Council for Foreign Medical Graduates (ECFMG). This exam was a prerequisite for coming to the United States for further training as a medical resident. The exam tested not only my medical knowledge but also my command of the English language.

I grew up immersed in English because my father, having been trained under the British system, insisted that we speak English at home in order to hone our skills. It was only with Amma that we spoke in our mother tongue of Telugu as she had not received an English education. To this day, I often speak with my siblings in English. Even when we do make an effort to speak Telugu to one another, English words find their way into the conversation.

Telugu is an ancient language with ninety-five million speakers worldwide, mostly in India. It dates back as far as 1500 B.C.E.. For comparison, English has only existed since around 1000 C.E.. There are twenty-two languages recognized in the constitution of India and contrary to what some believe, they are not dialects but distinct languages, most of which have their own unique lettering systems. Telugu has a fifty-six character alphabet and shares no characters at all with Hindi, the most widely spoken language in India. I speak and read both languages and additionally speak Urdu, which is an official language in both India and Pakistan.

Despite preparing me for it all my life, my father was disappointed at the prospect of my leaving India. Once I explained to him my reasons, including the incident with my examining professor, he understood enough to wish me well and see me on my way.

It was difficult to find a location where the test was offered because India was doing its best to discourage medical school graduates from leaving the homeland and practicing medicine in places like the United States. They were trying to prevent us from draining the "national brain trust."

This was understandable, especially given that India had subsidized our medical education. Unlike medical students in America, who often end up with mountains of student debt, I paid very little tuition at medical school. After investing so much in us, the government expected us to stay in India and be of service to the locals.

I was the top student in my medical school class and the second-highest scorer at the state level which included three medical schools. I was hardly the only defector, in fact, the top four or five students in my class as well as a plethora of others came to America.

When international flights were a luxury and even telephone communication to India was an expensive prospect, these classmates and I would get together as sort of substitute family. As we got older and started families of our own, our annual reunions provided my children with cousin-like relationships not yet available to them elsewhere.

Eventually, several of my siblings moved to America. Between that and the availability of flights abroad, I have been able to remain close to my birth family as well as my chosen one.

Because of the Indian government's attitude, the ECFMG test was not scheduled anywhere nearby so we had to go to Colombo, Ceylon (now known as Sri Lanka). To get there, I had to take an overnight train from my home in Hyderabad to Madras (now known as Chennai) followed by an hour-long flight to Colombo.

I successfully completed the exam in September of 1970. In June of 1971, after a compulsory internship in Hyderabad, I received my M.B.B.S degree from Osmania Medical College. An M.B.B.S, or Bachelor of Medicine / Bachelor of Surgery is the equivalent of an M.D. (Doctor of Medicine) degree in the United States.

Coming to America

My degree in hand, it was time for me to leave India and start my new life in the United States. It was July of 1971 and I was one month shy of my twenty-third birthday. There were no direct flights from Hyderabad at that time, so I needed to take a flight from Hyderabad to New Delhi, spend one night at a hotel, and then catch a flight from New Delhi to London followed by my final destination of Detroit, Michigan. Although I had done an internship before leaving India; as a foreign graduate, I was required to repeat the process stateside. I chose Highland Park General Hospital in Detroit for my second internship.

I said very emotional goodbyes to my family at the airport in Hyderabad. Although I was making a large leap forward in my life, it was quite sad for all of us. We were a very close-knit family, all ten of us, and my youngest sibling was only ten years old. I had never lived away from my family home before; my medical training so far had all taken place in Hyderabad. I remember the tears shining on Amma's face and the ones I tried to keep at bay. She gave me a hug, kissed my cheek and said, "Take care of yourself and keep in touch."

My father and I had always been very close but his demeanor was always more formal than my mother's. He had had some military training and enforced discipline sternly when necessary. That is not to say he was not a loving man but he definitely had his own way of showing it. As my siblings and I celebrated various accomplishments throughout our lives, we always knew our father was very proud of us even though he never said it directly. He was subtle and subdued in his manner. He expressed his affection through his eyes and his smile. Despite not hearing certain words from his lips, not one of us ever doubted for a moment that he loved and adored us. My father gave me his biggest loving smile and said, "Take care of yourself and remember what I taught you about taking care of your patients." I could see Nannagaru's emotions written all over his face. Like with my mother, I responded in kind

Once I got on the plane, I attempted to bury myself in a medical textbook to try and take my mind off the sadness I felt over leaving my beloved family and country behind. I thought about the words of my mother, reminding me to stay in touch. I would do my best, of course, but it would not be as easy as it sounded. In those days, placing a call from the United States to India was expensive and complicated. We were still decades away from cell phones and the whole system was much more basic. Any time I wanted to call home to India, I had to contact an operator to book the call. They would tell me that once they were able to connect to the party I was trying to reach, they would call me back. Sometimes it took half an hour to connect with my family, and each minute of the call cost four dollars!

The night before my 2:00 a.m. flight, I stayed at a hotel in New Delhi. Knowing I had an extremely early flight (or late, depending on your perspective) I requested a wake-up call from the hotel front desk. Unfortunately, The hotel staff failed to wake me at the appointed time. I managed to wake up on my own a little later than planned. Now running late, I got dressed as quickly as possible, ran out of the hotel, and hailed a taxi. I paid the driver extra money to take me to the airport as quickly as possible. There was no traffic at that hour, so we made good time to the airport.

I rushed inside the airport and sprinted to my gate. By the time I got there, my Pan Am flight had already boarded and the airplane door was closed. Fortunately, they still allowed me to board the plane. Security was very different in those days. I went through none of the processes we do today. In the current climate, I am sure that I would have missed the flight. Back then, however, I was able to hand off my baggage to airline personnel and board the plane.

I may have just been lucky, or it might have been thanks to my friend Chakri that I was able to catch that flight. A medical school classmate of mine, he had stayed at a different hotel the night before and had gotten to the airport in plenty of time. When I found Chakri in his seat on the plane, he told me that he had informed the flight staff that I was expected. That might have been a contributing factor to my being allowed onto the plane despite my late arrival. At this point, there is no way to know for sure.

Once we reached London, I had some time before catching my flight to America. The flight staff announced that any passenger on the connecting flight to America was welcome to stop over in London, at their own expense, of course! I did not want to miss the opportunity to spend a couple of days in London. I arrived on a Thursday and booked my final flight to Detroit for Saturday.

I was elated to have the chance to see London and grateful to be able to afford a ticket for the tour bus. Because Indian banks did not keep much U.S. currency on hand, they were only able to give me eight dollars in American money when I left India. I was fortunate that my brother Sudhakar worked in a bank, as he was able to get me another fifty dollars.

So, with a total of fifty-eight dollars in my pocket, I felt rich. That sum of money obviously went a lot further in 1971 than it does today. I used a bit of that money to tour London. I had some knowledge of English landmarks and knew the names of certain places I wished to visit, like Trafalgar Square. I spent a couple of days going all over London by bus, enjoying myself. On Saturday, I boarded the plane for the final leg of my journey.

My New Life in America

When I arrived in America, I had no idea how to get to the hospital where I would start my future. Thankfully, there was a fellow Indian resident-in-training who was familiar with America and able to assist me. He had been on the same flight I was and had been in the States before. It was very common in those days before cell phones and Uber rides for one Indian traveling abroad to help a fellow countryman looking lost. He explained that I should take a shuttle to the central bus station in Detroit, and take a cab from there to the hospital. It took the last of the money I had in my pocket to pay the cab driver. When I arrived at the hospital, I was completely broke. But I had arrived intact and with my luggage, so overall, my journey from India to America was smooth.

I had one last challenge when I arrived at Highland Park General Hospital. I was a scrawny young man and weighed no more than 135 pounds. I was struggling to get my heavy suitcase inside the hospital. Suddenly, a seven-foot-tall man appeared out of nowhere, towering over me. He had dark skin like mine but did not look Indian at all. He was the very first Black man I had ever set eyes on; he was a security guard at the hospital. The man picked up my suitcase as easily as if it was a cup of coffee and carried it inside for me. He was a friendly, wonderful man and was very helpful to me.

I had come a long way but at last, I was safe and sound at my destination. I now found myself in a country that was truly foreign to me in every way. From the moment I boarded that first flight in Hyderabad, I had begun to miss my parents and siblings. It was a very long and lonely flight and now that it had ended, I was stuck with an even more lonely feeling, knowing that my family was so far away.

Housing arrangements had been made for me as part of my internship. After announcing my arrival at the hospital and identifying myself to the staff, I was assigned to a two-bedroom apartment and given the door key and directions. My roommate was an intern at the same hospital. Although I started out shy, I soon made friends with other house officers (a term that encompasses interns, residents, and others in training). Little by little, the loneliness that had consumed me began to subside.

After my internship at Highland Park General Hospital, I continued my training with a residency in internal medicine at Sinai Hospital, also in Detroit, which I completed in 1974. Sinai Hospital provided excellent training to me as well as an introduction to the love of my life. It was there that one fateful day, I met a beautiful woman named Karen. A young student, she was working part time to save money for college. It was love at first sight for us both. She would soon become my wife.

Forty-six years and two grown children later, we are still happily married. Karen recently told our young grandson that when we met, I made eyes at her in the elevator. As precocious as Milo is, I am not sure he quite understood what it means to "make eyes at" a girl. Whether he did or not, he just smiled, accepting our love story, old fashioned phrases and all.

Karen enriches my life in so many ways and I love her dearly. She has been instrumental throughout my career in encouraging me to be involved in games and sports which help to offset the emotional impact of dealing with sickness and death every day of my working life. I got involved in tennis and later golf as enjoyable ways to ease my stress and was able to do so only with Karen's support in her care of our children, our home, and even my social calendar.

CHAPTER 5

Hanging Out My Shingle

Starting My Married Life

KAREN AND I met in 1973 and planned to get married in Detroit, Michigan in 1975. In early November of that year, I was on the phone with my father, talking to him about our wedding plans.

At first, my father did not want me to marry a girl so different from myself. Not only was she not of my caste, she was not even the same religion as us. We had a longstanding family tradition and by marrying Karen, I would be breaking it. I would be the first child in my family to marry a non-Indian, a non-Hindu, and even the first to marry a non-Brahmin spouse.

"Why don't you come to India later this month and get married in a Hindu ceremony here?" suggested my father.

This was a compromise of sorts. He would not object to me marrying Karen if we agreed to have a traditional Hindu ceremony. The bargain struck, we decided that the wedding was to take place around the time that Thanksgiving is celebrated in America.

I have to give my parents extraordinary credit for their open-mindedness. It was no small feat for both of them to overcome their resistance to me marrying someone so different than they had planned for me. Being welcoming to my choice of bride was a very liberal position for them to take, especially my father. In retrospect, I would have completely understood if he had voiced vehement objection to the union.

I gave no advance thought to what I would do if my parents objected to my choice to marry Karen. I believe that being raised with the habitual practice of acceptance served me well in this instance, as it has throughout my life. I knew that I would be able to accept whatever position my parents took regarding my marriage, and learn to live with it. So, there was no point in analyzing the situation or envisioning various scenarios in advance. As I cannot imagine my life without Karen, I am glad I never had to face that dilemma. I know that marrying despite family objections can be very hard on a young couple and was overjoyed not to have such an obstacle in front of us.

When I told Karen about my father's invitation to get married in India, she agreed even though it meant not having her own family present. My father arranged to have a Hindu priest marry us in a traditional ceremony. In mid-November, we made the long journey from Michigan to Hyderabad.

Within a few days of our arrival, my family got a call letting us know that my mother's mother, who lived about a hundred and fifty miles away, had suffered a stroke. She was only semi-conscious and the doctors did not expect her to survive long. It was a longstanding tradition that a wedding could not take place within fourteen days of a death in the family.

With my grandmother's death so imminent, our Indian wedding was canceled. I left Karen with my parents in Hyderabad and went to attend Ammamma (as I called my grandmother in Telugu). We had decided that, given the inevitable postponement of our wedding, Karen would return home to Michigan without me, and I would join her after my grandmother's funeral. When I arrived at Ammamma's home, I started her on intravenous fluids. She had lost her power of speech during the stroke and did not seem like she would live much longer when I took over her care. By the time I left to return to my parents' house however, she had begun showing signs of improvement. She had started moving and even attempting to speak.

With Ammamma on the mend, I returned to Detroit to reunite

with Karen and make plans for the wedding we would now be having. Meanwhile, my mother, being an only child, brought my grandmother to live with her and my father in Hyderabad. At that time, not only was it traditional and respectful to care for elders at home, but there were not really any nursing homes or assisted-living facilities in India, so it was practical and necessary as well.

On December 6th, 1975, Karen and I were wed in a simple ceremony at a Greek restaurant in Detroit, Michigan.. Our joining was presided over by a judge and followed no particular religious tradition. We were all very disappointed that my family was not able to be present at the wedding.

In lieu of my family, I invited eight friends of mine from Osmania Medical College who were now living in the States. They were like brothers to me and I was very grateful to have their attendance though I still missed my own family, of course. Although it has been over half a century now since we left school, I still talk to many of them on a weekly basis and participate in regular group Zoom calls. Our wedding was also attended by my new family; Karen's parents and four younger brothers.

Because of the time we took off to travel to India prior to our wedding, we were unable to take a proper honeymoon. I needed to get back to work and we consoled ourselves with the idea that our trip to India had been sort of a pre-wedding honeymoon of sorts.

In 1977, Karen and I took our first trip as a married couple to see my family in India. We rented a twenty-foot bus with a private tour guide / driver. We spent time with my family and visited some interesting historical sites. We returned to India many times, initially just for family weddings, but once our children were born we went more often, wanting them to be exposed to both their family and their culture. I have also traveled to India several times on my own and once with each of my children as my sole companion. I must say that international flights are much easier with a teenager than a five-year-old!

When our son and daughter came along in 1979 and 1983 respectively, we agreed to give them Indian names to help them stay connected with their Indian heritage despite growing up in America.

My name is reminiscent of my father's, which was Ramakrishna and I wanted to continue that tradition with my son. However, it was also important to us that our kids did not have names which would be unpronounceable to most Americans. As a compromise, we called our firstborn, Naveen Krishna. His first name is spelled phonetically enough that most Americans have little trouble with it. We had no way of knowing that a Disney Prince would be given the same moniker thirty years later! By continuing my family tradition in my son's middle name, something that was more common in America, we hoped to honor both sides of his heredity. By coincidence, we assigned the same initials to our daughter, Neena Kalyani. Her middle name does not come from a family member but does mean beautiful and auspicious in Sanskrit.

As for Ammamma, she lived for twenty years after her stroke. Until her eventual passing in 1995, she became ambulatory, first with a walking stick and then under her own power. Although she walked hunched over, she was able to move about and even contribute to the household by sorting grains and lentils before they were cooked for dinner.

This story about my grandmother perfectly illustrates the fact that even those who are considered experts in their field cannot always predict a person's life expectancy no matter what data they have. There are so many different factors that contribute to when, why, and to what extent certain people recover from potentially fatal medical events like strokes or late-stage cancer diagnoses and others do not. Science, while the best we have, only goes so far. That is one reason why I feel it is so inadvisable to give a specific life expectancy duration. As I grew and matured as a physician, I learned that lesson for myself.

As for my father, getting to know Karen as a person helped him quickly overcome his initial reservations about my choice of wife. Over the years, he became extremely fond of her. She even joked that it would be difficult for me to "get rid of her" now that she had my father's stamp of approval. The fact that we presented him with a grandson and granddaughter made him very happy. He loved all of his grandchildren very much. My father taught himself to use an old treadle sewing machine and made special Indian clothes for our children. For Neena, he made a traditional lengha, an Indian skirt and blouse outfit. For Naveen, he made a kurta set, which is a little bit like lounging pajamas.

Now, my father has passed on and I have my own grandchildren to dote upon. Milo and Kaia, they are the children of my son. Life comes full circle.

Dreaming of Making a Difference

During the last year of my residency, I had big ideas about my future. I dreamed of one day making a real difference in cancer research. Back in the 1970s, oncology as a specialty was still relatively new.

In 1974, I began my fellowship in oncology at Henry Ford Hospital in Detroit. Dr. Robert Talley, one of the founding members of the American Society of Clinical Oncology (ASCO) was chief of the division at that time. He was a fine teacher and a true gentleman, with the ideal personality for patient care. I learned the importance of compassion from the example set by both Dr. Talley and his associate, Dr. Robert O'Brien. Throughout my career, I tried to emulate the compassion these fine doctors showed to their patients.

My dream of making a difference in the field of cancer research led me to apply to the National Cancer Institute (NCI) in Bethesda, Maryland. After two interviews, I was offered a senior fellowship to begin in July of 1976, immediately after finishing my fellowship in oncology. In April of that year, not long before my fellowship was to begin, Karen and I rented an apartment in Silver Spring, a suburb of Bethesda with more affordable housing options for a young couple just starting out. Then, only two or three weeks before the start of my job, I received a call from NCI, rescinding their original offer and replacing it with one at a lower level. This call would change my life, as I later realized, for the better.

Instead of starting as a senior scientific officer, I would only be a junior scientific officer. As I was fully qualified for the original position, I found this change extremely disappointing. I had interviewed with

NCI twice, and was making plans to uproot my life and Karen's in order to work for them. Such a change at the eleventh-hour just felt wrong to me. I felt as though accepting it would send the wrong message to NCI and start my relationship with them on the wrong foot. So, I declined the offer and in doing so, found myself in a position where I had no idea what the future held for my career.

When I told Dr. Talley what had happened, he suggested that I join a Henry Ford Oncology alumnus who had gone into private practice across the state. Following his suggestion, I joined my colleague in his practice, and made Kalamazoo, Michigan my home. Karen and I ended up living there for thirty-five years. Both of our children were born and raised there.

I had a very satisfying professional life, learning from patients who showed exemplary courage through sickness and even in the face of death. I was fortunate to have the opportunity to train medical students and residents from Michigan State University and become the founding medical director of the West Michigan Cancer Center.

From time to time, I would hear from residents I had trained who were now in practice and seeking my input on a particularly difficult case. I always welcomed these calls. Interacting with former residents about their tough cases was always a fascinating endeavor. Occasionally, one of my former trainees would tell me that they had chosen to practice my own specialty of oncology thanks to our time together. It was very fulfilling to know I had made such an impact. I still receive letters from residents of decades past. The following is an excerpt from a letter I received after sharing an early draft of some chapters from this book.

> We have four kids. Our son... and our daughter-in-law... are going to give us our first grandchild (a boy!) in March. I spend my time reading, playing guitar, and am starting to pick up some rental properties to fix up and rent. I like to keep busy!

> *I loved your memoir thoughts. I want to spend some more time reflecting on your writings and will share more thoughts after I've had time to let this marinate a little!*
>
> *I, too, am playing with a memoir. I'm pulling together meaningful patient cases, be they clinical conundrums, medical mistakes, or diagnostic dilemmas that I've encountered along the way, and the life lessons I have learned from them. Some are funny, some are sad.*
>
> *I'll try to give you a call soon, maybe this weekend, though I'm on call for the Palliative Med service, so it all depends on how busy we are. Look forward to reconnecting soon.*

I treasure correspondence such as this, which reminds me of the impact I have had on those who worked with me and how their lives turned out.

CHAPTER 6

Impactful Life Lessons

My Father's Wisdom

Throughout my life, I have been fortunate to run across many different types of people who had tremendous positive influences in my life. I call them all my teachers. My very first teacher was my father. I have never forgotten the great advice he gave me when I received my acceptance letter to medical school.

I followed his advice throughout my long medical career, treating everyone with respect and compassion and giving my patients hope whenever possible without deviating from the truth. I have always strived to treat people as I wish to be treated. I would put myself in the proverbial shoes of my patients so that I could have empathy for them and better understand what they were going through.

In addition to the lesson that my father taught me as I was about to enter medical school, I also carry with me to this day additional wisdom that he shared. Some of these lessons deepened in meaning for me as I got older and experienced more of life.

My father was a disciplinarian and taught us that, above all things, we must always be honest and show compassion to our fellow human beings. He was a man of great character and taught all of us children that disposition and temperament can truly be everything.

"If you tell one lie," he taught us, "that will lead to you having to tell many more lies to cover it up."

Communication with a Purpose

Early in my professional career, I noticed that the majority of terminal cancer patients were able to accept their diagnosis and prognosis. The key was to make them aware of the reality of their situation, to explain their choices honestly and clearly, and to always involve them in the process by giving them options and hope. Patients are more satisfied with their care and tend to have greater acceptance of their illness when they are included in making the decisions about treatment options. I learned how to communicate more effectively by working with these terminal patients.

Giving patients the opportunity to express their concerns, fears, and hopes is also a critical part of helping them find acceptance of their illness. Studies have shown that, on average, doctors interrupt patients after eleven to eighteen seconds[12]. I found that a patient was better able to accept their illness when I let them speak without interruption. In fact, it took me less time to explain the details of their disease when I let them get their thoughts out first. Many patients at the end stages of their cancer confided to me that pain and suffering was of greater concern to them than death. Most of them were already aware of their status but were hesitant to open up about this to their family and friends.

As a patient came to accept their terminal prognosis, they were better able to help their family through the anger and disappointment they felt over losing a loved one. Cancer patients and families face physical, psychological, emotional, and financial challenges. The courage shown by these patients in spite of their challenges has been a continual source of inspiration for me as I fight my own cancer battle.

Again and again, I have learned the truth of the saying, "If you don't have your health, nothing else matters."

Kindness and Compassion

Both of my parents impressed upon all eight of us children the importance of being kind and compassionate to each other. I also learned a lasting lesson in kindness and compassion during my final year in medical school in India.

I was rotating through an eye hospital at the time. One day, in the outpatient clinic, I witnessed one of the greatest examples of kindness that I have ever seen in my life. It was a lesson I will never forget. Although it may not have been the best decision from a practical point of view, the man who made it did so with nothing but compassion in his heart.

A patient in his fifties came into the clinic with a towel wrapped around his right eye. He was thin and wore partially torn clothes and one of his slippers was held together by a pin. The attending physician uncovered the man's right eye by carefully removing the towel. The patient's entire eye was extremely swollen, nearly popping out of its socket. In India, exposure to intense sunlight is a common contributing cause of the development of cataracts at a relatively early age.

This patient was from a small village, thirty miles from the city where we were. This hospital offered medical services at no charge and would have been available to the patient as soon as he noticed an issue. Either the patient was unaware of the existence of this free eye hospital or could not afford the transportation into the city; possibly both.

Instead, he sought treatment from a local self-styled ophthalmologist, a barber by day. For generations, barbers have dealt with more than just hair; treating people with cataracts, toothaches, and other minor surgical concerns. Centuries earlier, someone had discovered a quick but very risky way to correct cataracts. It was this gruesome procedure that our patient had undergone at the hands of the barber-surgeon.

The treatment involved using a fine needle to push the opaque cataract lens through the cornea and into the vitreous humor (the back chamber of the eye). Once the cloudy lens was pushed away, patients would be able to see more clearly. The entire process took less than a minute. In 1969, the fee for this barbaric procedure was five rupees (or about eighty cents in American currency).

This procedure had a disastrous and predictable effect on the patient. The contaminated needle caused panophthalmitis, infection of the entire eye. The only treatment at that point was enucleation, or complete removal of the eye. During the British rule of India, couching, the procedure that had ruined the man's eye, was banned and punishable by a fine, payable to the victim.

The attending doctor under whom I was doing rotations in the hospital explained to the patient that we would have to remove the infected eye. Then, before removing the patient's eyeball, the doctor asked him to provide the name of the barber who had blinded him in one eye. The doctor explained that the patient was entitled to compensation. for his ordeal

The patient refused to identify the barber. In the local language, he said with a smile, "I will not tell his name. If he goes to jail, his wife and three children will go hungry. I can see with one eye just as good as with two."

Here was a man who could barely afford to eat two meals a day. Yet, he had an enormous heart, filled with compassion and concern, even for a man who had wronged him. I have never forgotten the lesson he taught me that day by example, a lesson about the true meaning and value of kindness and compassion.

I carried the lessons I had been taught about kindness and compassion into my practice as an oncologist. The following letters from patients of mine show how much of an impact kindness and compassion can have on patients who are suffering and afraid:

> I feel compelled to write you this note. I was devastated to hear that my CA-125 was going in the wrong direction and there were no further surgeries possible. I have never been so afraid in my life. I think I really faced death from cancer for the first time since I was diagnosed.
>
> I am feeling better now and thinking positively. I have come to grips with this. I am taking control of my thoughts and my body and will work with you to focus on beating this monster into submission.
>
> I am remembering what you said and am counting my blessings. Dr. Vemuri, you are one

of my special blessings. I value your wisdom, your judgment and your friendship. I know you are giving me the best care you possibly can. I am very blessed to be living in Kalamazoo and have the West Michigan Cancer Center staff available. Thank you for everything and most of all, for your understanding.

~ * ~ * ~

We are sure you know what a beacon of hope and optimism you have been for our entire family for the past nearly four years. We wanted to write to express our earnest gratitude for your consummate treatment of my husband and our father, John.

Thank you for exercising your vast knowledge and medical skill, which certainly prolonged his life considerably. More importantly, thank you for your ever insightful and compassionate treatment of the complete patient and family.

Thank you for being a friend to all of us and especially to John. You are a rare individual and a force for good in the universe. A visit with you became a source of strength for him, leaving him buoyed and girded for the struggle.

~ * ~ * ~

I have been trying to write this note for some time. Russ's illness took its toll on all of us. However, your caring and sincere manner somehow helped us to get through those last *days. I believe that you are not only an excellent doctor but also a kind and compassionate man.*

I can't thank you enough for everything you did for Russ and our family. You will always be in our prayers.

Surround Yourself with Beauty

A patient and friend named Diane taught me an important lesson about the value of surrounding ourselves with beauty. She was a phenomenal human being with courage, faith and spirituality.

I used to play golf with her husband, also a friend, and their son went to school with mine. In some ways, it was difficult to treat a patient with whose family I was so close. Diane's husband encouraged me to tell her story as an inspiration to others. He sent me a book with her poems and drawings she completed before her demise and gave me permission to share them. In this book you will find a few examples of her artistic talent: pictures drawn with her non-dominant hand and poetry which expresses her deepest thoughts.

When Diane first came to me for treatment in May of 1998, she was a fifty three-year-old woman with cancer of her right breast which had already spread to her liver and lungs. The swollen lymph glands in her right armpit were impinging on the nerves that controlled the function of her right arm, resulting in local paralysis and making it impossible for her to drive with her dominant hand.

Diane responded well to chemotherapy. She showed marked improvement in both her liver and lungs, with the disappearance of pleural fluid. Her right arm paralysis, however, did not improve and she was still unable to use her right arm to shift gears when she drove. So, when she returned to work as a teacher, her supportive husband drove her to school daily. He proved to be a great example of kindness, empathy and support. Diane herself exemplified so many wonderful qualities. She never let her illness stand in the way of her passion for creating art. Within a short time, she trained herself to use her left hand to draw exceptional pictures.

In addition to her love of drawing, Diane also wrote poetry. Here is one of her lovely poems:

> Look out the window
> Surround yourself with beauty
> Take in the sights
> Soar to new heights
> Erase the past
> Go step by step
> One day at a time
> Live in peace
> See the world
> Inside out

The following is an excerpt from Diane's memoir:

> My journey began in April of 1998 when I received a diagnosis of cancer of the breast, lung and liver. Along with chemotherapy, I also received six weeks of radiation. In July of 1999, I received good news that I was free of cancer in my breast and lungs. Three weeks later, I had problems with my balance.
>
> A CT scan revealed three tumors of the brain. Tumors on the nerves prevented all use of my right arm. Having been a totally right handed person and having dabbled in drawing twenty years earlier, I decided to draw using my only useful hand—my left hand. My journey is an ongoing passion for living.

Sadly, Diane died in December of 1999, after months of recurrence of cancer in her liver and lungs. Several of the pictures she drew with her left hand were still decorating the walls of the Cancer Center when I retired in 2011. She was, and remains today, an inspiration to me and many others.

She continued her positive message until the end. I will never forget her courage and the message of hope. She will always be one of my heroes. I am thankful to Diane's husband for letting me share his wife's story.

Detachment Without Indifference

During my many years practicing oncology, one of the most common questions I was asked by both physicians and non-medical people was, "How do you deal with being in a profession where your patients are facing death and dying on a regular basis?"

I understand why it could be hard for many people to fathom dealing with the sick and dying every day as part of one's profession. Yet despite this difficulty, I have no regrets. If I had to do it all over again, I would choose medicine, and specifically oncology, every time.

Early in my career, it became clear to me that witnessing sickness and death so constantly was affecting my quality of life; in particular, the quality of my sleep. Poor rest prevented me from giving my full attention and focus to my patients' problems. I knew that I could not continue on in such a manner.

I recalled the phrase "detachment without indifference" from the *Bhagavad Gita*. The most important part, of course, is to keep true to the "without indifference" part of the concept. I used this principle to formulate an approach to treating my patients that allowed me to continue to provide the best possible care to them without draining myself physically or emotionally. My belief in this teaching, and my practice of it, helped me to maintain my own inner strength during my many years as an oncologist and my many unfortunate patient losses.

It is important to remember that as human beings, we are not robots, and so can never completely master our thoughts, particularly the upsetting ones. With practice, however, one can keep their mind strong while remaining fully engaged with the daily challenges of life. I was able to develop a habit of keeping my brain from entertaining negative thoughts. I was able to do this as long as I knew I was providing the best possible care to my patients. I did not have to sacrifice my own well-being to provide for theirs.

An additional strategy to ensure that I was always able to maintain my inner strength and balance was to admit that I was not all-knowing or powerful. Any time I ran out of options to offer a patient, I would refer them to other care providers at major cancer centers with more expertise and experience than me. There is no room for hubris when it comes to people's lives. I applied this practice of detachment without indifference in my daily life as well and by using these techniques on a regular basis, I found that caring for sick and dying patients was less traumatic than before.

Unfortunately, in spite of providing the very best and latest treatments to my patients, some cancers just would not respond. For patients diagnosed with these types of cancers, death was an unfortunate but inevitable part of their prognoses. Every person is destined to one day leave this world. While all of us are aware of this fact, we do not always fully accept it and it is easy for a physician to feel guilty and question whether they did enough to preserve the life of a terminal patient.

By maintaining life balance, providing the best possible care, and referring a patient to more knowledgeable experts when necessary, guilt was reduced or even eliminated completely, since I could honestly tell myself I had done everything within my power. This is one of the secrets to my relatively stress-free and depression-free career caring for cancer patients.

CHAPTER 7

A Balancing Act

The Importance of Life Balance

I HAVE ALWAYS MADE it a priority to take care of myself both physically and emotionally. This may sound selfish but was essential in preventing burnout and enabling me to continually provide the level of care my patients deserved. Part of that care necessarily involved projecting a positive, upbeat attitude; something I could not have done if I had been constantly exhausted and emotionally drained by failing to maintain my own well-being.

I recall reading an article in a medical journal several years ago. Unfortunately, I do not remember the title and rely on my memory alone for the content. The article reminded me of the importance of preventing or reducing burnout while maintaining one's personal life, interestingly enough, by focusing on the alternative. The author, a physician and husband of a woman with terminal pancreatic cancer, described the extraordinary care his wife received in the final weeks leading up to her death. Her oncologist, fresh out of his fellowship training, would spend hours holding her hand and crying with her. The patient's husband was filled with gratitude and praise for the oncologist and his dedication.

The dedication of this man went so far as to keep him from enjoying other aspects of his life due to the guilt it made him feel for doing so while his patients were suffering. Apparently, this oncologist went to such an extreme as to avoid listening to music while driving to work lest he experience pleasure for himself. There is no question that he deserves credit for such extraordinary kindness and compassion. However, I have to wonder where that doctor is now if he continued to approach each dying patient in this manner, denying his own needs for self-care. This sort of behavior, while laudable, often leads to burnout and even mental health problems, which benefit nobody in the end.

There is a saying, which I have seen attributed to various sources, along the lines of, "Don't set yourself on fire just to keep somebody warm." This is similar to the directive we are given before every airplane flight; if oxygen masks are necessary, affix your own before aiding your children or others. Of course, obeying this does not mean that we love ourselves more than our traveling companions. The simple fact is that without the mask, the responsible party might pass out, therefore leaving their dependents helpless. Or, given the adage above, if you burn, what do those you helped do next? Self-care is becoming more acceptable to schedule and prioritize although there are still those who will not take time to attend to their own interests for fear of being thought selfish or cruel. As a society, we need to destigmatize this practice in order for those with difficult jobs or other responsibilities to survive.

Maintaining My Own Balance

I personally believe that all human beings, regardless of their profession, can benefit from having balance in their lives. In fact, I believe that such balance is not only helpful but vital.

The way that I accomplished this balance throughout my years as a practicing oncologist is the same way that I do today, as a cancer patient myself!

As previously mentioned, I have a long history of practicing detachment without indifference as prescribed by The *Gita*. Additionally, a huge part of my self-care revolves around staying active. As a young physician, I started by playing tennis and badminton on my off weekends in order to recharge my proverbial batteries. Eventually, I followed the example of many in my profession and took up golf as well.

When the mobile phone came into regular usage in society, I became able to play the games and sports I enjoyed even on weekends when I was on call since the technology allowed me to provide an immediate response to any patient who called with an emergency. My wife was always very supportive and encouraged me to play. In fact, without her abilities regarding our home life and childcare, I may not have been able to enjoy such freedom.

What constitutes life balance will vary widely for different people. For me, spirituality, meditation, listening to music, playing tennis, golf, and other games made me able to continue doing a difficult job while I was in practice. These activities continue to help me maintain my life balance today, even though the scales have shifted a bit in regards to my time commitments in retirement, I have found a renewed need to maintain doing the things that I love as I wage my own personal battle against cancer. This attitude has allowed me to remain calm throughout the twists and turns in my own medical journey.

There are more options than I could possibly imagine that people might use to maintain balance in their own lives. In addition to those I practice; reading, writing, travel, crafting, volunteer work, and video games are only a few that spring to mind. Everyone must find their own methods for achieving and maintaining life balance. The activities and hobbies that keep us energized, prevent burnout, maintain inner peace, and prevent depression and despondency will vary greatly and we have to remember that what works for someone else in our life may not be the hobby for us. For example, my wife is a quilter, which is something that does not appeal to me at all. Likewise, she has no interest in setting foot on a golf course. So, we spend time together doing activities we both enjoy and time apart pursuing our own interests.

It does not matter how you go about maintaining your own life balance, provided that it is something that does not interfere in the happiness of others, of course, only that you do so. Recharging one's own emotional and physical batteries prevents burnout. It also ensures that those we love and serve in both our professional and personal lives get to interact with us at our best.

To me, the spiritual aspect of maintaining my balance is every bit as essential as any other. Spirituality can go hand in hand with religion or be a completely separate concept. It just depends upon one's point of view. The following is a letter from a patient, acknowledging the importance of spirituality in the practice of medicine:

> I read that you will be a participant in "Spirituality in the Practice of Medicine: an uncommon conversation on incorporating personal spirituality in a healthcare setting." I am so glad this topic will be offered. Spirituality is the one component lacking in our managed medicine.
>
> You and I have met twice—once when my mother was dying. At that visit, you supported our decisions. Then we met again when I consulted you after my fourth cancer. Both of these meetings were life changing and contributed as much to our family healing as any other medical procedure.
>
> I had excellent technical expertise for my cancer treatment, but you saw me as a whole person—not a patient. I consider my recuperation to be a result of my conversation with you rather than my six-week post-op session with my surgeon. You removed fear and anxiety by treating me as a complete human being and not just a cancer patient. And your wisdom has allowed me to put the cancer behind me.
>
> Everyone knows that a patient at peace will heal faster and have less chance of a relapse. Thank you so very much for your gift of spiritual healing as well as physical healing. I am so glad

you will be sharing your expertise with other leaders.

The Impact of Attitude on Cancer

One thing I observed over and over during my many years as a practicing oncologist was how a patient's state of mind could impact their overall well-being, including their physical state. While it is difficult to draw a direct cause-and-effect correlation between attitudes and cancer, there is plenty of experiential and anecdotal evidence that a positive outlook and a healthy state of mind are essential in battling cancer and ensuring a better quality of life while doing so.

The American Cancer Society has a helpful support section titled "Coping and Living Well During Cancer Treatment"[13] which provides many resources to help those with the disease and their loved ones navigate the practical and emotional issues that come with a diagnosis. Among the articles on this page, is one entitled "Impact of Attitudes and Feelings on Cancer" which perfectly captures some of the questions that my own patients grappled with on a regular basis. It lists the following questions a person might find themselves thinking when told that they have cancer:

- *Did I bring the cancer on myself?*
- *Can having a positive attitude improve my chance of my cancer being cured?*
- *Can support groups and counseling help me live longer?*
- *Can I control the cancer by focusing on how my body is fighting the cancer or by thinking myself well?*

Of course, there are no universal answers to many of these questions but the article provides responses based on the current research. For example, while there are no data which show support groups and the like actually prolong life, there are still many benefits to participating in them, for example reducing tension and fatigue. While the quantity of life may not be increased, the quality of life certainly can be.

Likewise, there is no evidence that practicing mindfulness and guided imagery, as is commonly encouraged for cancer patients, has any effect on life expectancy. What it can affect, however, is the severity of certain symptoms including not only psychological issues such as anxiety and depression, but physical ones as well for some patients, such as nausea and pain.

The more that a patient is able to recognize and communicate their emotions and feelings, the more they are able to seek treatment, which often improves interpersonal relationships as well with caregivers and others who are impacted by their diagnosis.

Overall, despite the caveat that nothing attitude-related has been shown to make a cancer patient live longer, there seems to be plenty of evidence that maintaining the right attitude can make a cancer patient live better.

Maintaining a Positive Outlook, Despite My Diagnosis

I want to emphasize the power of positive thinking, even in the most dire of circumstances. Now I have the ability to speak about positive thinking and the importance of maintaining an optimistic attitude from the vantage point of a cancer patient, one I never expected to have for myself.

When I was diagnosed with metastatic lung cancer, I faced the challenge and the opportunity to refine and focus the same positive thinking practices I had used all my life; to in fact "practice what I preach" so to speak. I also had the chance to test many of the principles of Hindu wisdom with which I had been raised and which formed the basis of my spiritual and philosophical belief system.

As an oncologist, I know that my medical situation is precarious. I am not in denial about the likely course of this cancer. I also know that I am powerless to alter the inevitable outcome. While I can read and understand the latest research to an extent most cancer patients cannot, I still have no more control over the course of my stage IV non-small-cell lung cancer than any other person might. I do my best to stay calm regarding things I cannot control whether it be my cancer, the

COVID-19 pandemic, currently raging around the world, or any other disaster that might be coming my way. What I can control is my own reaction to catastrophic events, and the way I choose to deal with them.

Being both a cancer patient and an oncologist, I am able to be directly involved in my own treatment and to understand the choices and decisions I need to make along the way. One important aspect of my treatment is the maintenance of a calm and balanced state of mind. Thankfully, by the time of my diagnosis, I had already developed a daily practice which helps me in balancing both my mind and body.

I started doing this early in my oncology career when I was having difficulty dealing with the sickness and death I witnessed on a regular basis. I found that by remembering the lessons and wisdom from the *Bhagavad Gita*, the spiritual text I have continuously drawn from since I was a boy, I was able to develop a system for managing the more upsetting aspects of my chosen profession.

I trained my brain to approach the treatment of my terminal patients with detachment (meaning not letting it affect me) without indifference (meaning I still cared). I was able to apply that same practice in my reaction to my own diagnosis. This lifelong habit of detachment without indifference is what enabled me to hear my diagnosis and accept it without becoming angry or depressed.

Unlike many cancer patients, I have not had significant sleeplessness associated with the stress of my condition. In fact, with the exception of when I took Dexamethasone, for which it is a known side effect, I have not had any trouble sleeping at all.

I have an optimistic attitude because I choose to and I choose to maintain it every day. I have already exceeded my expectations for the course of my cancer. I will continue treatment and look forward to (hopefully) enjoying a good quality of life for years to come.

Physician Burnout, Depression and Suicide

The medical information site *Medscape* maintains an annual report regarding physician burnout, depression, and suicide in the US.[14] The 2019 report was both revealing and very discouraging. This article was based on responses from around 15,000 physicians in about thirty specialties. I was shocked and disappointed to learn that physicians have the highest suicide rate of any profession. What a sad thought that those we entrust to protect and save our lives have nobody to do the same for them. Reports of physician burnout and depression appear to be skyrocketing during the COVID-19 crisis that has been raging for nearly two years at this point but the true effects may not even yet be fully understood.

As an oncologist who enjoyed great career and personal satisfaction, I feel a responsibility to share with my fellow physicians some of my secrets for a highly fulfilling professional life. I believe my techniques apply to those not in the field of medicine as well.

I am well aware that physicians are practicing in a different medical climate than I enjoyed before I retired. When I started practicing oncology in 1976, I was working alongside a truly dedicated, compassionate and well-trained hematologist/oncologist in private practice. He was a wonderful human being and also happened to be a deacon at the local Baptist church. I was lucky to be practicing in an era when physicians were spared from some of the challenges they currently face including the bureaucracy of insurance and pharmaceutical companies.

Nevertheless, I had my own challenges during my career. As I've mentioned here, dealing with patients with advanced malignancies and poor prognoses on a regular basis was stressful, especially during the early part of my career. Dealing with younger patients was especially upsetting, to the point where it was affecting my sleep and therefore my quality of life.

Patients and their families carry an extraordinary burden and face multiple challenges after a cancer diagnosis. I knew that I needed to have a strategy for ensuring that I put forth a positive attitude and always provided hope to my patients. I realized how difficult it could be to stay positive and offer hope while also remaining fully engaged with patients' problems. It had become evident that feeling too much empathy could easily depress me. That is when I began to understand the necessity of keeping myself physically and emotionally strong in order to provide the best care for my patients. I discovered that I was best able to provide hope and a positive message to them when I took good care of myself.

Doctors must put their self care before their care for their patients. This translates to better doctor-patient relationships and more satisfied patients, often even healthier patients! Putting one's own self first may sound selfish yet it is necessary for the survival of everybody involved.

CHAPTER 8

Challenges

The Challenge of Electronic Medical Records

ONE OF THE challenges faced by many physicians in practice today is the increased role of bureaucracy in medicine. Many physicians these days (including my personal internist) are required by the hospitals that employ them to see a certain number of patients per hour. This removes the physicians' freedom to provide adequate care, as they were trained to do and as would be best for the patients. This leads to dissatisfaction and frustration for both doctors and those under their care.

An issue that surprises many people is that of electronic medical records. In theory, they seem like something that would make the lives of doctor's easier but it turns out that is not always the case. Several physicians I have spoken to, especially the older ones, are critical of the complexity of electronic medical records. A few physicians in their early-to-mid sixties retired earlier than they had planned, due to the complexity of this method of record keeping.

Fortune Magazine highlighted this problem in an article entitled "Death By A Thousand Clicks"[15] which was critical of the government for spending thirty-six billion dollars on what is considered by many to be a failed digital revolution. The variety of record systems and their sometime lack of compatibility can have fatal consequences.

Challenges Facing Cancer Patients
Complications from Cancer Treatment
There are many challenges which cancer patients and their oncologists face when trying to determine the best course of cancer treatment to pursue. One of the most challenging aspects of these decisions involves the complications that can arise from treatment. Every treatment has side effects and those must be considered before moving forward with any particular treatment plan.

The best way to make such decisions is for oncologists to involve not only the patients but also their spouses and families and anybody else who is a member of their core support system. As a team, they can weigh the benefits of treatment against the possible complications.

In some cases, they may also be weighing the benefits of receiving treatment at all against the idea of foregoing it altogether. The importance of quantity of life vs. quality of life varies and is a very personal decision. Keeping the patient and their family involved in all decisions gives the patient an important sense of control and keeps them hopeful.

Depending upon the type of cancer, the stage to which it has progressed, and a myriad of other factors, patients and their doctors may conclude that the complications and side effects are minor (or at least manageable) when compared to the potential benefit of treatment. There are also cases where the patient's diagnosis does not lend itself to treatment and even treatments where there is a significant chance of decreasing life expectancy. There are reasons to decide for or against each of these and only when the risks and benefits are fully understood can the patient feel good about making such a choice.

When patients do undergo chemotherapy, radiation therapy or immunotherapy, they may face any of a long list of side effects, depending on a number of factors including the specific medication and their body's response to it. This list includes (but is not limited to):

- anemia
- appetite loss

- bleeding and bruising
- constipation
- delirium
- diarrhea
- edema
- fatigue
- fertility issues (or later fertility issues in young patients)
- flu or flu-like symptoms
- hair loss
- infection and neutropenia (low white blood cells called neutrophils which can leave a patient susceptible to infection)
- lymphedema
- memory and/or concentration problems
- mouth and throat problems
- nausea and vomiting
- nerve problems
- organ related inflammation
- pain
- sexual health issues in men and women
- skin and nail changes
- sleep problems and insomnia
- urinary and bladder problems.

Complications and side effects can range from so mild as to be barely noticeable to so extreme that they do not seem worth the benefit of the therapy. Every patient will have their own individual response to their treatment plan. There is no way to determine in advance which side effects or complications a patient might experience. Patients should, of course, discuss all side effects and complications with their doctors before beginning any course of treatment.

The best way to approach treatment is to arm the patient with as much information as possible so that they can be prepared for any side effects and complications that might arise. It is also critical for patients to create a strong support network to help them cope during treatment.

Additionally, cancer support groups have been very beneficial to many patients by providing them with the support of other people who have gone through, or are currently undergoing, treatment for the same type of cancer. Even if they cannot expect the exact same results or effects, it can be incredibly helpful to know that they are not alone.

Delayed Effects of Cancer Treatments

Patients can sometimes experience delayed complications from cancer treatments; effects that may be felt years after the treatment is complete. Such delayed effects can result from any type of cancer treatment. This list of possibilities is as long as the list of immediate complications above and of course varies by therapy type. Of course these lists are in no way exhaustive.

After radiation therapy, delayed effects would depend on the location of the treatment site and may include:

- tooth decay and cavities
- early menopause,
- hypothyroidism
- heart and blood vessel problems
- increased risk of other cancers (for example, breast cancer) after mediastinal radiation for Hodgkin Disease
- infertility
- lymphedema
- memory and cognitive problems (after radiation to the brain)
- lung problems

Challenges

After chemotherapy, delayed effects may include:

- early menopause
- infertility
- dental problems
- osteoporosis
- heart problems caused by Adriamycin, Daunorubicin, Herceptin, or Osimertinib
- lung problems including fibrosis (scar tissue) caused by Bleomycin, arsenic trioxide (Trisenox), or Idarubicin (Idamycin)
- hearing loss caused by Cisplatin
- nerve damage
- peripheral neuropathy, a common side effect from chemotherapy with Cisplatin or Taxanes
- cognitive impairment, also commonly known as "chemo brain." For most patients, mental symptoms last a short time. For others, symptoms may persist for longer periods. Although attributed to chemotherapy, certain symptoms may be present even before chemotherapy is given. The theory is that cancer itself produces some cytokines (a chemical byproduct). There is also the fact that cancer patients are surviving longer and therefore, cognitive dysfunction can be seen. Exercise may improve cognitive processes.
- chemotherapy-induced secondary cancer

After hormonal therapy, delayed effects may include:

- blood clots
- hot flashes (in both women and men)
- increased risk of second cancers

- menopausal symptoms
- osteoporosis
- infertility
- impotence
- sexual problems

One common problem following hormone therapy in postmenopausal women is vaginal dryness and painful sex. In women with H/O estrogen positive breast cancer, the use of estrogen is contraindicated, even for topical applications. The decision as to whether or not to use estrogen despite the risks is a quality of life issue and can really only be made by the patient herself. I had just a few patients who decided to accept the risk of hormonal replacement many years after breast cancer without recurrence. The patients who did choose to use hormonal replacements did so only after a discussion of the pros and cons with their own physicians.

The decision regarding whether to use vaginal estrogen should be made in coordination with a woman's oncologist and gynecologist. It is important to note the committee opinion developed by the American College of Obstetricians and Gynecologists in March of 2016. They concluded that for hormone-sensitive cancers, there are safety concerns, even with topical estrogen. Non-hormonal approaches are the first-line choices for managing urogenital symptoms whenever possible.

Financial Toxicity

Cancer can have a serious financial impact on patients, just as on many other aspects of their life. Seeing this happen again and again, I came to think of it as financial toxicity. There can be various components of this financial toxicity. Of course a major factor of this is that the cost of cancer medication has increased exponentially over the years. Even those with medical insurance often pay very high copays which add up quickly, especially when multiple drugs are required.

I knew about these high costs but did not personally experience them until fairly recently when I went to the pharmacy to pick up my target therapy cancer medication. Despite the excellent drug plan of my health insurance, a thirty-day supply cost me $3,051 for the first month, and close to $1,000 each month thereafter!

According to one study by the *American Journal of Medicine*[16], 42% of cancer patients with a new diagnosis exhausted their life savings in just two years. Considering the cost of my own medication, I can easily see how this could happen, especially since pharmaceuticals are only a fraction of the many costs incurred by patients and their families.

The costs of all kinds of medication in the United States have skyrocketed and show no indication of returning to remotely reasonable levels. The entire situation is completely out of control for not just cancer patients but those with long term issues requiring constant supplies of medication such as epinephrine and insulin as well. Of course, my personal experience is with cancer patients, many of whom I have seen in terrible situations such as having to decide between paying for their medication and other basic necessities such as rent or food. Per a study by the Fred Hutchinson Cancer Research Center[17], people diagnosed with cancer are more than 2.5 times as likely to declare bankruptcy than the average American. Rates are even worse for younger patients who were bankrupted at up to ten times the standard rate.

Additionally, it is not uncommon for cancer patients to lose their jobs because they are too ill to work. This leads to increased financial hardship from both decreased income and loss of insurance coverage. Those patients who are without a support system for both financial and caregiving needs are hit especially hard by such a loss. Although resources are available for financial aid, there is never enough to go around and older patients often lack the technological literacy to pursue these opportunities online.

The WMCC, where I was the founding medical director, was aware of these issues. We employed financial counselors on site to be a part of our patient support services. These counselors would contact pharmaceutical companies in search of lower-cost or no-cost medications for our patients. Of course, the pharmaceutical companies we contacted would request detailed financial data from the patients before agreeing to provide any assistance and our counselors would help patients to understand the requirements and gather the necessary documents.

Another cost, often overlooked in the focus on pricey chemotherapy, is that of pain medication. While the palliative care provided by painkillers may not actually fight the disease in question, it can be invaluable when it comes to allowing patients to remain comfortable enough to have the strength to battle their life-threatening illnesses. Occasionally, I stepped in personally to provide financial assistance to patients who could not otherwise afford such care and I am certain there are other oncologists who do the same, knowing how important quality of life is to suffering patients. I hope to be able to continue to do so in perpetuity by directing all proceeds from the sale of this book to assisting patients who are unable to bear the cost of cancer treatments.

Impact on Family & Relationships

Any major diagnosis, including one of cancer, has a significant impact on the family and loved ones of the cancer patient as well as those with more secondary relationships such as co-workers and other associates. When a diagnosis is first made, the patient must contend with the shock of such news. Then, they must share the upsetting news with their loved ones and try to help them process their emotions, often before even having time to fully process how they feel about it themself, as the most impacted party. Just as the cancer patient needs hope in order to manage during treatment, their family and loved ones need hope, as well.

The emotional impact upon family and loved ones of a cancer patient is even more extreme when the patient has advanced-stage cancer. As a patient reaches the end stages of their disease, they must grapple with their own mortality at the same time they seek to put their affairs in order and seek to accomplish end-of-life goals. They may also feel responsible for reassuring those around them, even at the cost of their own emotional well-being. During this time, family and loved ones might be involved in assisting the patient with paperwork and other final arrangements even as they are processing their own grief and sadness over the inevitable loss to come. In short, it is not an easy time for anybody involved.

In addition to the emotional impact of cancer on the cancer patient and loved ones, there are more tangible factors such as the financial impact if the breadwinner of the family is unable to work due to illness or caregiving responsibilities. In this case, difficult decisions must be made as to how to continue to support the family throughout treatment and recovery.

This can put additional stress on a marriage. For example, if the spouse of a patient is unaccustomed to working and must start a job to help make ends meet, this can be frustrating, especially with limited earning potential due to being out of the workforce for a time. It can also put stress on the family dynamic, requiring one partner to bear the brunt of household chores on top of a full time job when the other is unable to contribute in either way. Funds initially earmarked for savings or allotted for other purposes must often be redirected toward the cost of treatment and/or replacement insurance coverage. As previously discussed, the cost of treatment can be astronomical and therefore a burden on the entire family.

Having open and candid conversations, starting at the time of diagnosis and continuing throughout the course of the illness, treatment, and sometimes slow recovery, can help a cancer patient manage the impact of the disease with their family and loved ones. It is helpful to address each emotional and practical concern and task as they arise, as opposed to letting issues and possibly resentment fester unaddressed, getting more difficult to resolve with each passing day. In this way, the patient and their family and loved ones can avoid becoming overwhelmed by a mountain of tasks and concerns that have piled up.

Lastly, it is important to remember that there are numerous resources that can be found online or through most cancer treatment facilities to help manage the varied aspects and impacts of cancer, both for the cancer patient and for their loved ones.

Talking with A Cancer Patient

It is easy to understand why it is important for anybody to keep open lines of communication with a cancer patient in their life. Even when uncertain about the best way to start a difficult conversation, it is necessary to press ahead. It can be awkward and uncomfortable to bring up such a painful and difficult subject and many may be tempted to shy away from approaching a loved one with cancer to initiate the discussion.

As *Cancer.Net* (a site maintained by the ASCO) notes in their section on Coping with Cancer[18], "It is better to say, 'I don't know what to say' than to stop calling or visiting out of fear." This shows acknowledgement of the difficulty the patient is in rather than avoiding the topic altogether. Taking care to show sensitivity is key in approaching a difficult conversation with confidence. Letting the patient lead the discussion and taking cues from them as to how much they want to talk about their situation and in how much depth is key to helping them feel comfortable discussing such an awkward and often depressing topic. Making an effort to remain hopeful and positive is one of the best gifts that can be given to a loved one with cancer, although that is not to say that unrealistic positivity is always helpful.

Taking care with phrasing will undoubtedly be appreciated by a cancer patient overwhelmed with negative thoughts. It is best to avoid making statements that could be construed as intrusive, blunt, or dismissive.

The following are some conversation prompts suggested by the site:

- I'm sorry this happened to you.
- If you ever feel like talking, I'm here to listen.
- What are you thinking of doing, and how can I help?
- I care about you.
- I'm thinking of you.

Conversely, the following statements are specifically listed as being unhelpful, some may come as surprising since they might seem empathetic but if considered from the patient's viewpoint, it is understandable how they could be harmful:

- I know just how you feel.
- I know just what you should do.
- I know someone who had the exact same diagnosis.
- I'm sure you'll be fine.
- Don't worry.
- How long do you have?

Showing love and support to someone dealing with cancer does not always have to involve conversation. Just the caring presence of someone who truly cares can be an invaluable show of support in and of itself. Being willing to listen and be present for a cancer patient is a gift, they may just want to talk through options, fears, hopes, or some combination thereof. The aforementioned site recommends that when talking with someone who has cancer, "Keep eye contact, listen attentively and avoid distractions when talking." Also, talk about other topics as well, not everything in the patient's life has to be cancer-related, after all! Sometimes what patients want more than anything is a taste of normalcy in their lives. A close friend or family member is ideal to provide that, since medical personnel definitely cannot.

Finding Social Support and Information

It is essential for cancer patients and their families and loved ones to surround themselves with support and arm themselves with information. The site Cancer.Net has a number of resources and recommendations for support at their website:

https://www.cancer.net/coping-with-cancer/finding-social-support-and-information

Topics at this site include:

- Counseling
- Finding a support buddy
- Telephone and email cancer helplines
- Support groups
- Online communities for support
- Wish fulfillment organizations for people with cancer
- International information for patients from across the globe
- Cancer-specific resources
- Government agencies

This is just one site and there are many more like it. The internet is an invaluable resource for support and information made easily available to cancer patients, their families and loved ones.

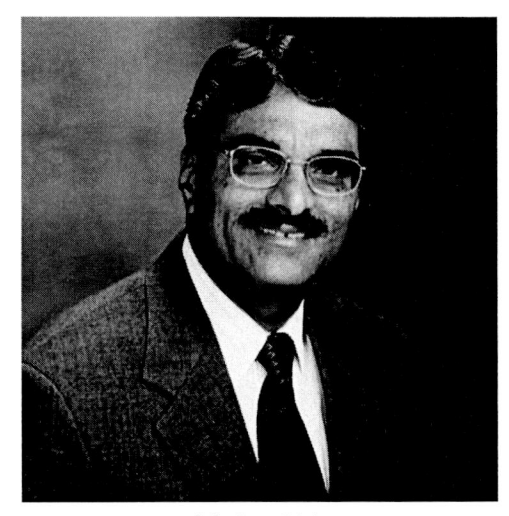

Me in 1994,
the year the Cancer Center was founded

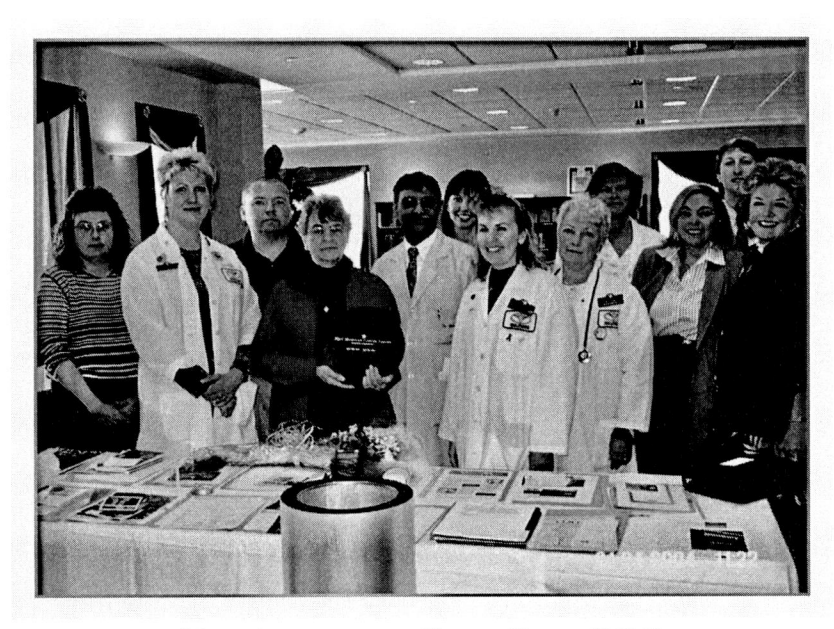

My retirement party, Cancer Center (2011)

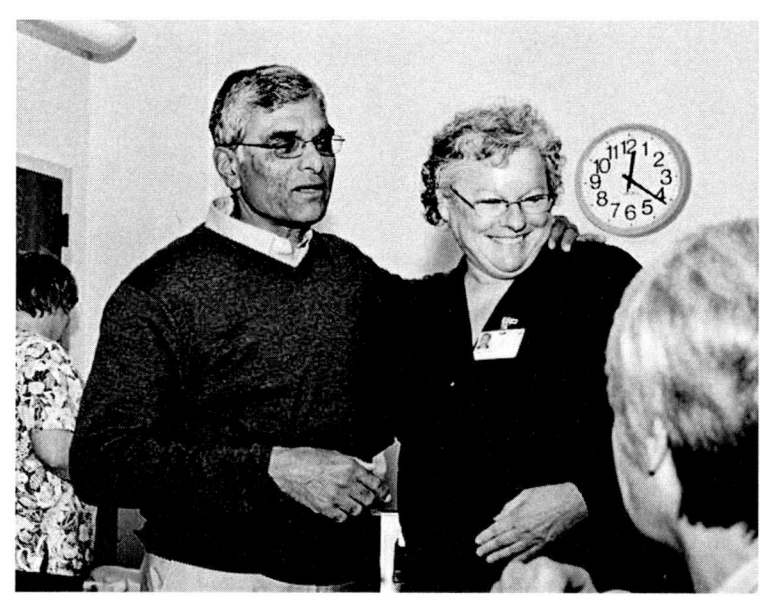

Me with a research nurse at the Cancer Center

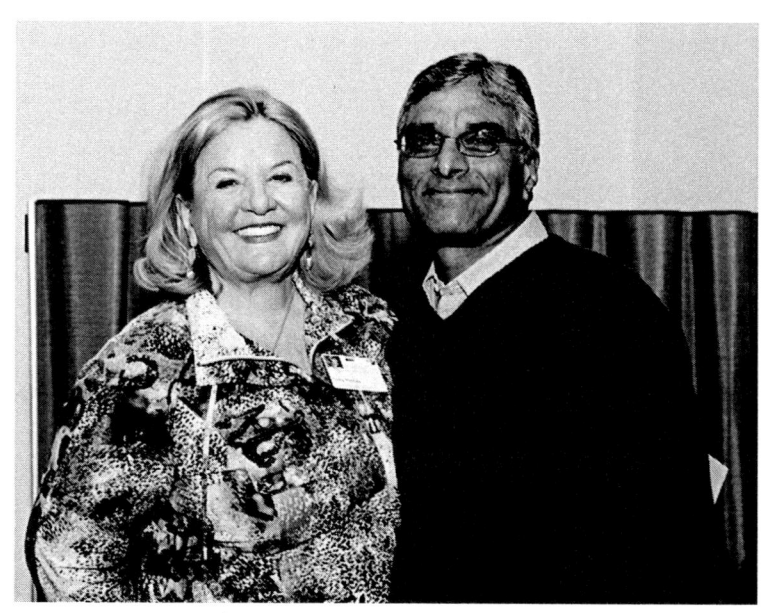

Me with Terry McKay, CEO, Cancer Center

Patient Diane's artwork and poems

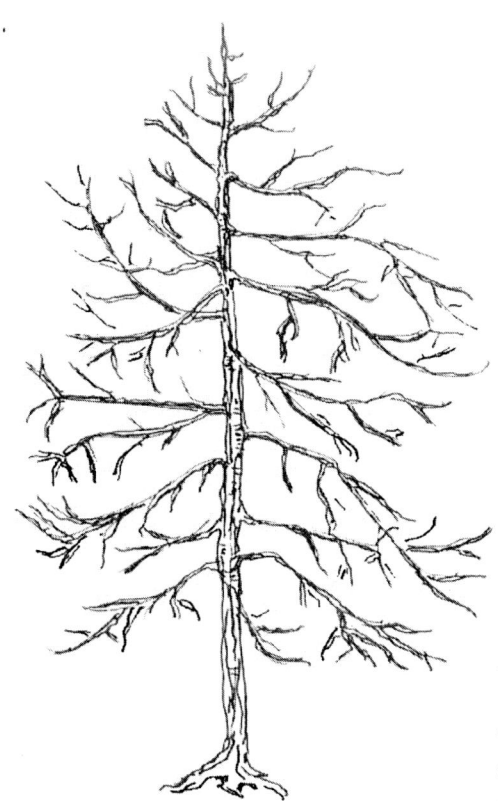

The Wisdom of the Tree

The wisdom of the tree
Can be seen in you and me –
we anchor, take root,
grow, through all seasons
learning, trying, growing
Then comes fall – an active time
we use to prepare
for the long winter ahead
to use what we know –
to be guided through
another year, and then we begin
all over again –
    Spring is that new beginning
    a time to renew

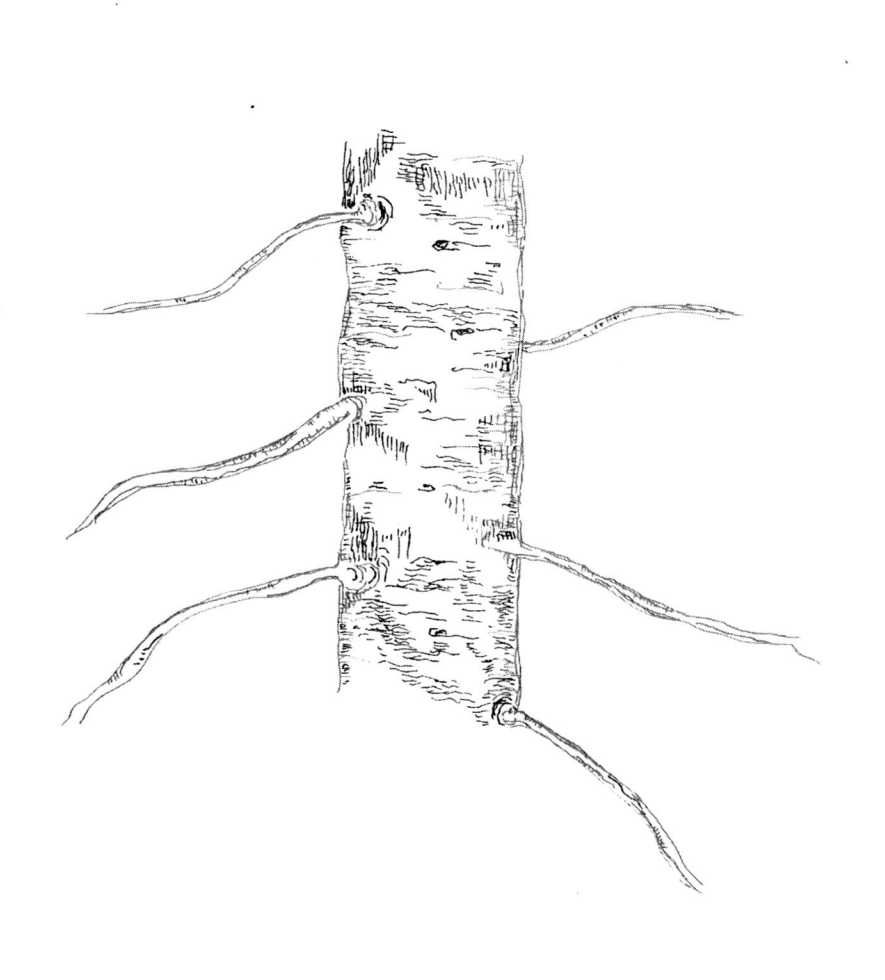

What Happens to You

It was a somber day when they
told you the truth.
You wanted to but couldn't listen
to what they had to say.
It didn't sound like it was for you
but for someone else.
The words seemed written, prescribed,
rather matter-of-fact, but how
would you rather hear it—
like buttered toast coated
with honey, cinnamon, and sugar
or plain and straight up?
Well, that's the way you got it.
Now digest it—there weren't rules
for that either, but you had
no choice except to let
the words come through for you
and do with them as you wish—
turn them around, say them back
to yourself any way you'd like
to hear them—know that timelines
are divine. You have a choice
in what you think, see and do.
Whatever is in store for you,
know that you have a choice too.

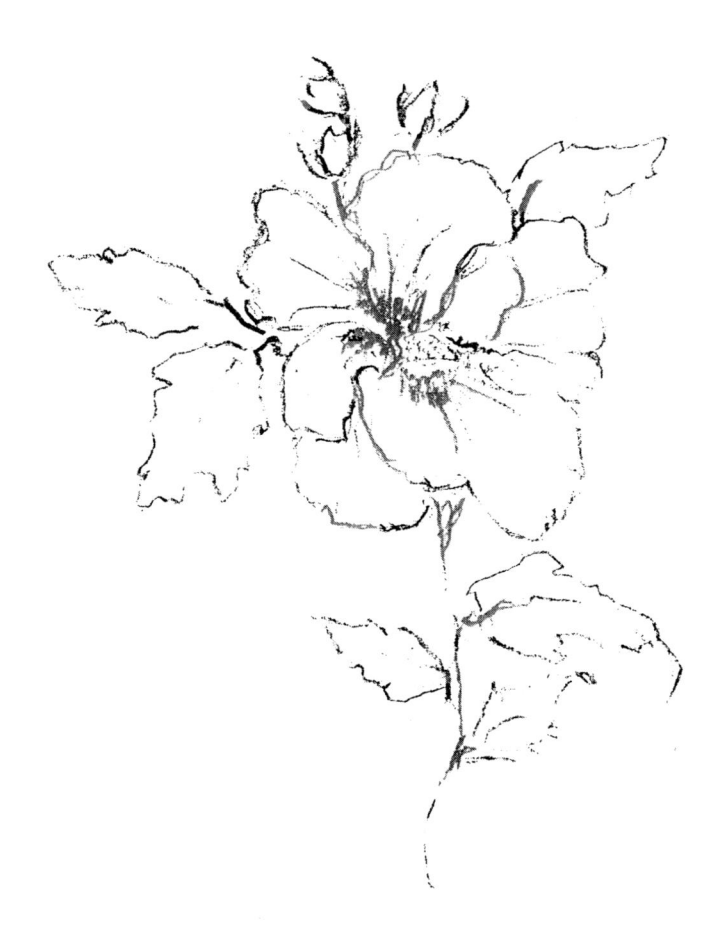

Insight 2

Let sadness come in
Let joy too be present with you
One does not diminish the other
One accepts each for the role they play
Each letting the other come and go
Not banning one in favor of the other
Each plays a tune, works itself out,
embracing all—that we think,
see and do
They reflect that which we've done
and that which we can do
Staying in the moment, practicing
what we know, sharing with
those for whom we care
Opening the heart, growing inside,
loving each part
Knowing we are part of the
Master Plan
Not to judge *why me*, but *what do
I do next*
Making each moment a new day
and saying "I love me in all ways"

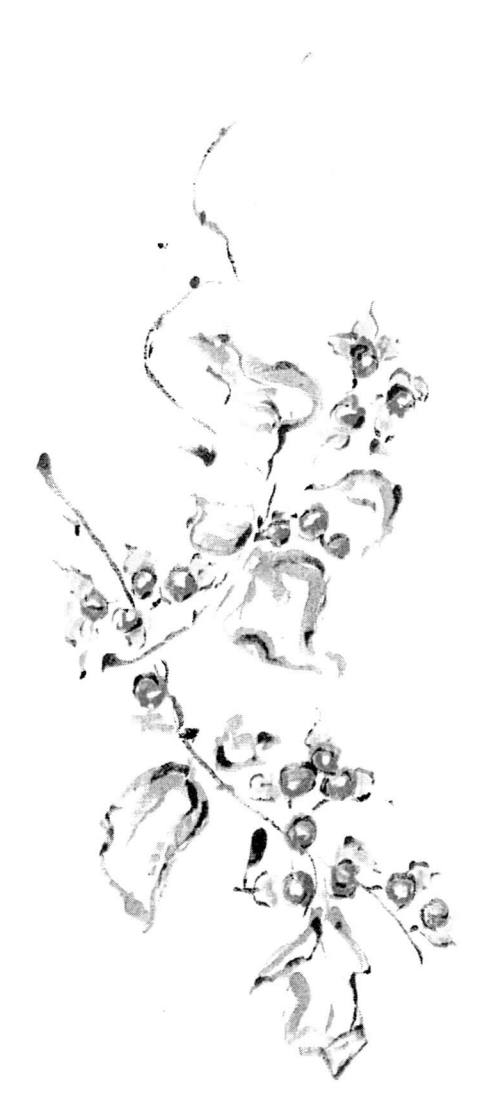

Untitled

With a song in my heart
    Peace on my lips
      Joy within
Thank God for who I am

The Wheel of Life

    A circle
Divided into segments,
Parts,
Each making up the whole,
That's life.
Parts, pieces, endings,
New beginnings,
Like a clock
Round
Made up of time/minutes/seconds
Parts of the whole
Parts that go on and on
That never stop
Only keep going/on-going/never an end.

    Life is a circle
Of which we're made up
Of all the lives of the past
And of the future yet to come

Remember, you're made up of parts
Of more than one
That's what makes you
That wonderful being
Who you really are

One within
Divine
No surprises
No compromise
Just as life is
Simply a circle

Trees

The seeds they sow are the souls

The wind that jostles about spreads life

We are seeds not yet grown

With miles to go, winds do blow

Seeds sown

We reach the end only

To be sown again

Spread by the wind

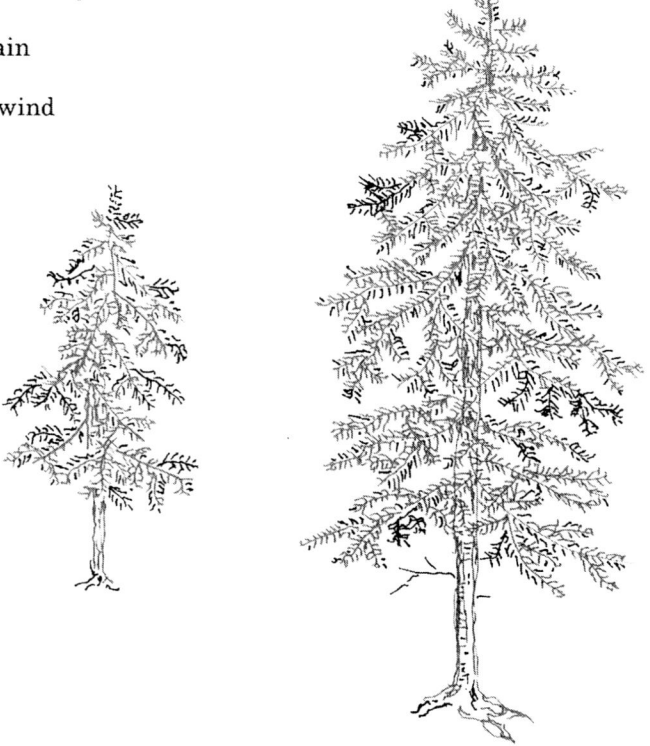

No Hair

No hair
not an issue—
see yourself as sexy
having more time,
time to do what makes
you happy

Laugh inside, clear out debris
Reach the outer dimension—
carefree laughter, let joy
come through, it tickles
you inside, can't hide,
makes others around you happy too

5/22/99

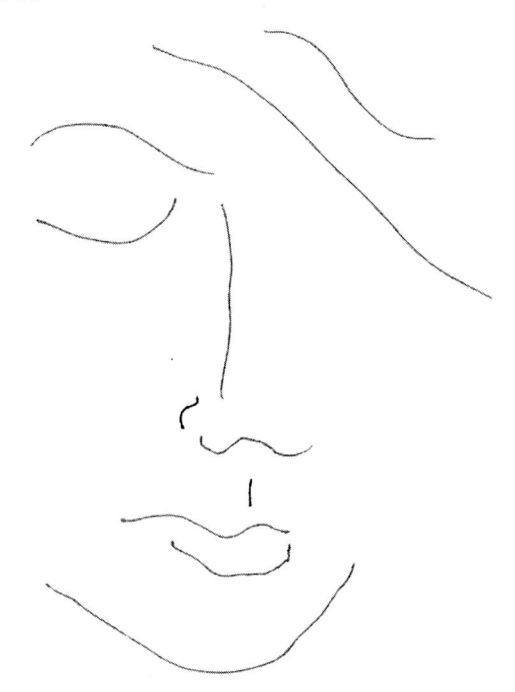

It is in the twilight

we see the light

In the dawn we see

the sunset

It is the bridge

of time between

that has meaning.

Bring peace within

for all time.

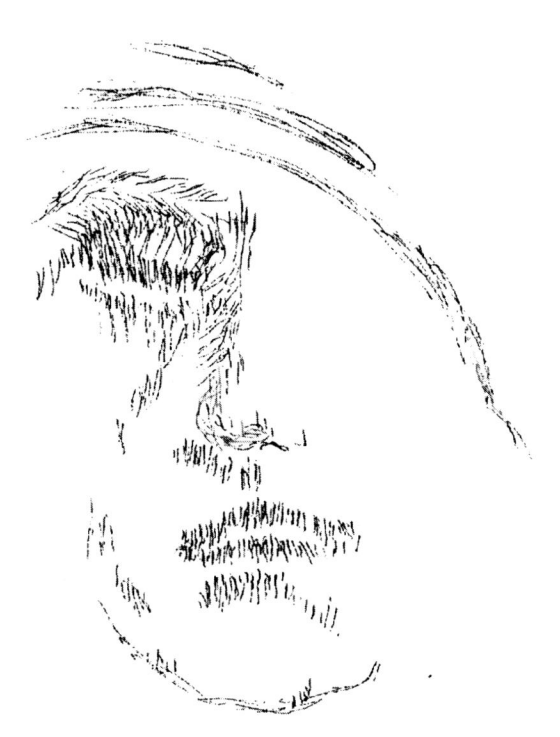

Keys
Thoughts are feelings
Felt physically in the body
Under every feeling is a definite emotion
Under every emotion is a definite perception
The Key –
Change perception
Change emotion
Feeling and Thought
About the Situation

CHAPTER 9

When the Truth is Not Enough

Hope Despite A Dire Prognosis

WHEN MARY, THE sixty-three-year-old woman who came to me for a second opinion regarding her dire pancreatic cancer prognosis, first arrived in my office, she made a lasting impression on me. I entered the exam room for our initial consultation and saw her seated beside her husband. He was tenderly holding her left hand, and had his right arm around her shoulder as Mary was wiping away her tears.

I introduced myself and asked, "What brings you to my office today?"

My question triggered a cascade of tears. Mary became so overcome with emotion, she could not recover her composure for several minutes. Once Mary had calmed down a bit, her husband spoke up, "We are here for a second opinion. The specialist we saw earlier said my wife has a life expectancy of only four months or less!"

Having already reviewed Mary's medical records, I knew that she had pancreatic cancer which had metastasized to her liver.

"When we saw the first oncologist," Mary explained, "I watched him going over my medical records on the computer. At one point, he read something that made his expression totally change. He started shaking his head. It was easy to tell that whatever he saw was negative."

Her husband, John, had asked the oncologist, "What is the concern, doctor?"

Averting his eyes from the computer screen, the oncologist had told the couple, "I'm sorry to tell you this but the prognosis does not look good. A CT scan shows fairly extensive involvement of the liver."

"I was frightened by his words," explained Mary, "and John was frustrated."

John said that he "asked the doctor what he meant by poor prognosis, and he said, 'With such extensive liver involvement, her life expectancy is four to six months.'"

"What the doctor was telling us seemed unreal, and I went numb," said Mary. "Before I realized what was happening, John pulled me up from my chair and led me out of the exam room."

The following day, I had a chance to talk to Mary's original oncologist and get his side of the story. He was sincere and explained to me that he had only given her the truth in regard to her life expectancy. While I could not disagree with his projection of a four-to-six-month life expectancy based on statistics, I doubt that I would have presented the information to Mary and John in the same manner. I would never lie to a patient but there are times when the truth alone is not enough. I felt that this was one of them.

I believe there were two essential elements missing from the way this oncologist presented Mary's life expectancy to the couple. First, he volunteered it before either had asked the specific question. Some people do not want to know how long they might live or are not ready for the information yet. There was no reason for him to introduce what sounded to them like a death sentence with so little preamble. Second, he did not take the time to develop a rapport with his patient and her husband. Because of this, he was basically a stranger giving them the worst news of their lives and not somebody with whom they felt they could discuss options for treatment and palliative care. In fact, they were not presented with any options at all before being given the dire information.

Sometimes Comfort is A Patient's Best Hope

Unfortunately a seemingly nihilistic approach from medical professionals, like that in Mary's case, is all too common. With such an aggressive malignancy and poor prognosis, knowledgeable people looking at her information would know there was nothing that could be done to alter the outcome. Although the prognosis was accurate and sincerely provided, when it is delivered in such a way as it was to Mary, it can completely rob the patient (and by extension their loved ones) of any sort of hope. This means that the patient is not presented with their options in an environment which is conducive to understanding and deliberation so they can feel as though there are no options at all, which can be the most devastating of realizations.

Fyodor Dostoevsky once said, "To live without hope is to cease to live." As both an oncologist and a cancer patient myself, I could not agree more with this sentiment. I believe that it is our responsibility as oncologists to provide hope, even if only in small measure, and to do so without being unrealistic or deviating from the facts. Hope can come in many forms and, as I have stated, encompasses far more than the singular goal of becoming cancer-free. Even if the response rate to a particular treatment is small, a patient and their support system should be part of the decision whether or not to pursue it. A doctor who has seen this before may think that the chance of benefit, slim though it is, would not be worth the possible detriment of the treatment. Alternately, they may think that any hope of prolonging life should be encouraged regardless of the toll it could take on the quality of life a patient has remaining. Either way, it is important that a physician present the options, including any available clinical trials and/or experimental treatments, and let the patient make the ultimate decision. Empowerment can be a beneficial treatment of its own.

I am sure that my colleague felt he was doing the right thing when he delivered the truth to Mary about her prognosis. In fact, his estimate regarding Mary's life expectancy turned out to be quite accurate. I cannot say that his approach was wrong, precisely, so much as incomplete.

Now that Mary was my patient, I explained to her and her husband about the chemotherapy options for her cancer, and the expected response rates. I also discussed side effects with them and explained that there could be an option to enroll in a clinical trial. In her particular case, the benefits of any treatment would be minimal while the side effects would likely be significant and severe. The kind of life-and-death decision Mary was facing could not be made without all of the information and a full discussion of her options.

Mary and John asked me many questions about what she could expect in terms of pain and quality of life if she chose to opt out of chemotherapy. After I talked to them about the availability of hospice and palliative care to keep her as comfortable as possible, the couple wanted time to fully consider their decision.

I assured them that they were welcome to take all the time they needed to decide, and left them alone in the exam room. Less than half an hour later, Mary and John came to a decision to forego chemotherapy.

Personally, I felt that Mary had made the best choice for herself but if I had told her that from the beginning, it might have affected her thought process.. "Tell me," I said, "why did you come to the decision to decline treatment?"

Mary's husband explained that they were scared by the thought of chemotherapy: such terrible side effects and no real chance of a cure.

"What is your hope now?" I asked Mary.

"Being kept comfortable and free of pain," she admitted..

For Mary, her only hope was for comfort, which she could only accept once she realized that a cure was an unrealistic goal. As I have previously stated, hope for cancer patients comes in many forms. We must always adapt hope to the individual patient.

Mary felt comfortable with her options and experienced a good quality of life. She chose palliative and hospice care to keep her free from suffering. Within three months, she passed away, surrounded by her loving family.

Her case reminded me of an important truth: every word an oncologist says to a patient matters. If we are not careful, a single word can take away what hope they have remaining.

Over the years, I had many terminal cancer patients like Mary. They all seemed to have a hunch that a true cure was not a realistic option for them. During one-on-one discussions with such patients, they often expressed their wish to be kept comfortable with as little pain as possible. Comfort was the definition of hope for these types of patients.

Interviews with 120 terminal cancer patients revealed that their most common concerns were not only regarding physical issues but rather spiritual, emotional, and family issues as well. This shows that medicine alone is not enough to fully treat such patients.[19]

A Prescription for Reducing Guilt

When a patient opts to receive no treatment, it can leave the surviving spouse and family with terrible feelings of guilt for letting their loved one die, even when there is nothing they could possibly do to change the outcome. This is, of course, not necessarily a logical feeling. Even when the treatment being considered has an extremely low chance of success, for example, one percent, the patient's surviving family can still experience tremendous guilt that it was not attempted. I have personally witnessed many families living with such unfounded and unnecessary guilt.

They can be plagued by questions such as, "What if our loved one had taken the treatment? Would she have lived? Was there more that we could or should have done?"

By including the patient's support system, including their spouse and family in the discussion about options and the ultimate decision, there is less likelihood that the survivors will struggle with guilt or even anger. By being involved, they can better understand the reasoning of a patient for choosing to "leave" them instead of fighting until the very end for only the tiniest chance of prolonged life - sometimes a life in which they cannot interact with loved ones anyway.

Eventually, I established an approach to help reduce or alleviate guilt on the part of the families. Any time one of my cancer patients told me that their son, daughter, spouse, or some other member of the family was strongly encouraging them to take a treatment that they had decided not to pursue, I would say, "Why don't you invite the whole family to join you in my office? They can all ask their own questions."

Having the entire family assembled in my office enabled them to be included in the treatment decisions being made by their loved one. Even if they were not directly involved in making the decisions, just being present for the conversation about treatment options was effective. This approach helped the family feel like they had made crucial decisions as a team. I found that this approach helped reduce the guilt and resentment the family felt after the passing of their loved one.

I was often asked by a patient or family member, "What if it was somebody in your family who had this type of cancer and was trying to decide whether to go ahead and get this treatment? What would you advise them?"

My answer was always the same, "I have no double standards. My recommendation would not change, even if it was a member of my own family."

Later in life when my father was diagnosed with terminal cancer, I was given the opportunity to prove the truth of what I had been saying all those years. I did not look at my father's cancer differently, nor even my own decades later. I followed the same advice I have given countless others.

The Power of Condolences

During my years in practice, I had a habit of sending condolence letters to the surviving spouse and family when a patient of mine expired. In these letters, I would highlight the patient's virtues and what I got to know about them while they were still alive. The following response I got is indicative of just how much this can mean to the family afterward:

> Thank you for taking the time in your busy schedule to express your heartfelt condolences to me and my family at the death of Marjorie. She indeed showed courage in spite of knowing the outcome.

At our first family meeting with you at the Cancer Center, we both told you about praying to God for a good doctor and competent nurses. You especially were the answer to our prayers. Thank you for caring. God bless you as you help and encourage others.

Healing with Good Humor

Despite my good intentions in sending out condolence letters, I have also committed my share of mistakes. There is one error in particular which always brings a smile to my face. My secretary would check the obituary column of the local newspaper and give me the names of those who passed away over the weekend. I would use this information to send my condolence letters.

I sent one such note to the wife of a patient who had suffered an unexpected demise. It turned out that I was not the only one surprised by this patient's sudden death. During my office hours later that week, the allegedly deceased patient showed up in person to present the condolence letter to me, saying, "Doc, you're killing me before my time!"

Needless to say, I was caught off guard and extremely embarrassed by my gaffe. Apparently, there was someone from our town of the same name and approximate age and my secretary had no way of knowing they were not the same man. I apologized profusely for my mistake, knowing that receiving such a letter could be both confusing and upsetting to a living patient. Fortunately for me, my patient was more inclined to see the comedy than tragedy in the situation, allowing my mistake to have no consequences beyond my own embarrassment.

This was one of the many advantages of maintaining a good patient-doctor relationship. We could each cut each other a bit of slack and ultimately, I learned from my mistake, taking more care to verify the identities of those listed in the obituaries before contacting patients' families!

CHAPTER 10

The Three Categories of Patients

Category One: Cureable

IN MY DECADES as a practicing oncologist, I came to think of my patients as falling into three different categories.

The first category was patients who were cureable.. These patients were fortunate to have their cancer completely cured, whether by surgery, chemotherapy, radiation, immunotherapy or some combination of those modalities, or they were in remission with a high probability of becoming completely cancer-free.

As I have repeatedly stated, hope for patients does not always include a cure although, of course, some patients are fortunate enough for that to be a possible outcome. Even in the most hopeful of cases, however, I would never promise anyone a cure. Instead, when a patient presented with early-stage cancer for which there were effective remedies available, I would only tell them that there was a possibility of a cure.

I was careful not to promise a cure because with cancer, one never really knows. Every body is different and reacts uniquely to even the most proven of treatments. Therefore, it is not right or fair to state definitively that a person will be cured. Being excessively optimistic when it comes to cancer can result in giving patients a false sense of hope. Being careful not to promise a cure which is not guaranteed is just as important as being careful not to take away hope by stating a definite life expectancy to terminal patients.

From the beginning of my career in the specialty in 1976 and throughout the decades in which I was a practicing oncologist, I always followed the same approach: I provided the facts with compassion and hope without ever compromising the truth or deviating from reality.

Periodically,, I received a letter from a patient, letting me know that they appreciated my approach. The following is one of those letters:

> Thank you from the bottom of my heart for all that you have done for me over the years. Not only did you take care of me but my dad and brother as well.
>
> You told me on the day we met that I might expect to live ten years with the cancer I had and then maybe have to look at a bone-marrow transplant. My initial bone-marrow transplant orientation meeting was ten years and two months after my initial diagnosis.
>
> Today I am cancer free. My transplant was four years and ten months ago. I am so thankful to you for taking care of me and helping me see the birth of my two granddaughters and see my younger son get married this year. Thanks again for all your work, care and compassion.

Category Two: "Not as Bad as I Thought"

The second category was patients with metastatic disease who had no realistic chance of a cure but could do well with long-term maintenance treatments. These patients also had the hope of future treatments being developed in the event of a malignancy recurrence.

This category of patients often reported to me that the experience of undergoing treatment was "not as bad as I thought it would be." In these cases, the patients could live their lives with reasonable normality and handle their treatments much like patients with other chronic illnesses such as diabetes or kidney disease.

I received the following letter from the family of a patient who, at the time of the letter, was doing well and living a full life:

> I received your lovely letter a few weeks ago and wanted to tell you how very much your words touched my heart. Robert is doing well and is teaching physics, part time. He did suffer a "widow maker" a few summers ago but has bounced back amazingly.
>
> Since 2004 when you treated Robert for head and neck cancer, he discovered that he had prostate cancer. In 2007, he received radioactive seed therapy. On the 23rd of this month, Robert will celebrate his 76th birthday.
>
> This would not have been possible without you. Thank you! Thank you! Thank you! My heart will always be filled with gratitude for the excellent care you extended to Robert fifteen years ago.
>
> You not only gave him a chance to raise his beautiful daughter, Kate, but gave her a lifetime hero—you, the doctor who saved her father's life! Today, Kate is pursuing that dream and plans to attend medical school. One day, she will be saving lives like you did. You ignited a fire and a passion in a little girl that continues to burn brightly today.

Category Three: "Easier Than I Thought"

The third category was patients who had either exhausted all treatment options, had widely metastatic cancer with significant comorbidities not suitable for any further therapy, or late stage cancer which had gone untreated for some time before they were diagnosed.. Many of these patients talked to me about the process of dying.

I remember visiting Beverly, a patient of mine, at Rose Arbor, an inpatient hospice facility in Kalamazoo. During one of our conversations, she told me, "This is easier than I thought it would be." She was one of many patients who expressed that same sentiment.

After Beverly passed, I received a letter from her family. Here is an excerpt:

> *Thank you for your wonderful condolence letter! Beverly showed us courage, hope, patience, perseverance and love for life. She seemed to be at peace with herself.*

Most of my late-stage cancer patients were aware of their dire prognosis but not necessarily a realistic life expectancy. I constantly saw disappointment on the faces of these patients and their families at the end stages of the patients' lives. Thanks to the honest and compassionate, although difficult, discussions I always had with my patients, I never experienced overt anger as a result of a patient's suffering or passing. This includes angry letters from patients or surviving family members, which I know some physicians have received.

The following are excerpts of actual letters I received from families of patients of mine after the death of their loved ones. I feel that these letter excerpts perfectly illustrate the fact that these end-stage cancer patients valued comfort above all else. They each had certain unfinished things they wanted to accomplish before they passed and wanted to be kept comfortable enough to accomplish those things. These letters also show the appreciation the families felt, knowing their loved ones were comfortable and sharp enough to take care of their end-of-life tasks.

Thank you for guiding Mother through her transition. Your caring attitude gave her assurance that she needed to face life with courage and her ver-present sense of humor until the end.

~ * ~ * ~ * ~

Thank you for exercising your knowledge and medical skills which certainly prolonged his life considerably. More importantly, thank you for insightful and compassionate treatment of both patient and family.

~ * ~ * ~ * ~

Thank you for being a friend to all of us, especially to John. A visit to your office became a source of strength for him, making it easier to face the struggle.

~ * ~ * ~ * ~

Thank you and your staff for five years of caring for Julia. You gave her the hope she needed to carry on until the end. Even when she was told that nothing more could be done, she was able to absorb it and come to terms with it.

Julia remembered your statement that the definition of hope may change over time. Having her stay in [in-patient] hospice until the end gave her that hope of comfort.

~ * ~ * ~ * ~

Thank you for being such a special person in Hank's life. He always spoke so kindly of you and appreciated your professional and personal attention.

He was able to make something for all the grandkids for Christmas. He even made one last toy for our two-year-old granddaughter on her birthday. You will always be remembered by me as a doctor who went the extra mile and made Hank's care special.

~ * ~ * ~ * ~

I personally want to thank you for all the love, support, concern, and helpfulness you showered upon my dear, dear friend, Norma. Yesterday near 4:30 p.m., Norma left her earthly home to be united with her mother and others gone before. It was God's will and he knew best. Her suffering was done.

We have wonderful memories of thirty-three years of friendship, which will be our treasured possessions.

Both Ron and Norma were so very comfortable with you, as well as their son . . . and their daughters . . . and daughter-in-law . . . I was so pleased that when it came time for Norma to have an oncologist, they chose and got you. I'd spoken of you to them so often.

Norma always knew her time on earth was limited after her diagnosis but she lived it to the fullest. Her main dreams were to see her niece get married, her granddaughter graduate from grade school, and her grandson play his sport.

Again, thank you from the bottom of my heart for your support and encouragement.

~ * ~ * ~ * ~

We want to thank you for the care and support you gave our mom. She thought a lot of you. She was a very gutsy lady but now she's in a better place.

~ * ~ * ~ * ~

Finally, I am able to fulfill Marshall's wish to show you this photo taken while he was in the service in India. He was such a virile, strong twenty two-year-old, full of hopes and dreams. I have now spent two lonely years without him, after 49 wonderful years with him. Cancer just doesn't play fair!

Thank you again for your kindness while he was in your care. He thought of you as a friend as well as his doctor.

To a large extent, these letters are a tribute to the wonderful staff with whom I worked at the West Michigan Cancer Center. Having them to help organize, oversee and facilitate the services we offered our patients ensured that the patients were pleased and comfortable prior to their passing, even when it was inevitable and seemed too soon.

We always told our patients the truth, communicated with them thoroughly and with compassion, made sure that they understood what was transpiring, kept them informed about the state of their health and the options to address it, and provided support throughout their treatment. These things made all the difference in their satisfaction level. We were fortunate to have excelent staff like Terry and Barbara to oversee, organize, and supervice the WMCC.

The Question of Life Expectancy

I always invited my patients to ask me any questions they might have, and allowed them to speak without interruption. I found such consideration to be the first step in gaining their confidence. One of the questions I heard the most often was, "How long do I have to live, Doctor?"

Most oncologists, once they have practiced even a short while, have become quite familiar with that question. Thanks to the widespread availability of medical sites online, of varying quality and reliability, many patients have some idea of their prognosis. Of course, the ideas that they get from searching the internet may be far from accurate. Even when their information is gleaned from the more trustworthy sites, not all factors may be considered or even understood by the patient or loved ones looking for answers online.

Every oncologist is familiar with the statistical survival data for metastatic diseases and we all know that life expectancy can vary greatly depending upon the primary cancer. I realized early in my career that it is ill-advised to quote a specific life expectancy, even from legitimate medical literature when still early in the treatment process.

In fact, I had a personal policy of not predicting a fixed number for life expectancy unless dealing with advanced cancers after exhausting all reasonable treatment options.

When a doctor gives a set number of months or years for life expectancy, the patient often hears only that number and forgets everything else the doctor has told them. The predicted life expectancy number can haunt the patient, having a terribly negative impact on their quality of life. This can turn into frustration if the number turns out to be incorrect whether the patient lives a longer or shorter time than initially predicted.

One patient told me, "Once I heard the number of months I had left to live from my previous oncologist, it became difficult for me to maintain my quality of life. I have trouble sleeping. In the middle of the night after using the restroom, I try to fall back asleep but I can't. The thought of dying in six months keeps me awake at night!"

Therefore, I took great care with the way I answered the question, "How long do I have to live, Doctor?" I would explain that the range is an average and may not apply to every patient. With newer treatment options, your prognosis can be much better than the average! This is especially true when applied to the more treatable cancers, such as breast cancer, papillary thyroid cancer, lymphomas, testicular cancer, etc.

If a patient demanded their life expectancy in order to plan for the future, I always felt it was appropriate to provide the answer this way: "That is the statistical average for your particular cancer but keep in mind that you could be an outlier."

The caveat about any patient possibly being an outlier was important. By wording my answer in that way, I was able to be completely honest without taking away the patient's hope through dire predictions or what might sound like an absolute. Years later, I find that I am happy to be an outlier myself, having survived my own cancer far longer than the statistical average predicted at the time of my original diagnosis.

CHAPTER 11

Case Histories

Linda: Beating the Odds

In April of 2005, forty two-year-old Linda came to me for a consultation regarding her metastatic breast cancer. I will never forget the frightened expression on her face when we first met. A biopsy had confirmed breast cancer, grade 2/3, indicating that it was moderately aggressive. Understandably, both Linda and her husband were extremely anxious. Like many people, they believed that a diagnosis of cancer was the equivalent of a death sentence.

A whole-body CT scan had revealed multiple spots on Linda's liver, strongly suggestive of metastasis. A bone scan showed increased activity in her lower spine and numerous ribs where she had growing pain meaning the cancer had likely spread to her bones as well.

Tests revealed Linda's cancer to be estrogen/progesterone positive, meaning that her cancer was feeding on those hormones. Linda's HER-2 (human epidermal growth-factor receptor 2) test was negative. This was a good sign because a positive HER-2 test generally indicates a more aggressive cancer.

The message I gave to Linda and her husband was, "Even though I don't expect that you will be 'cured,' hope is not lost. Hope for you involves improving both your quality and quantity of life, with the help of the latest treatments already approved by the FDA."

Knowing that Linda's cancer was estrogen/progesterone positive had therapeutic implications since she was premenopausal. However, I gave her chemotherapy instead of an antihormonal (estrogen blocker) treatment like Tamoxifen. The two cycles of Doxorubicin and Taxol which I prescribed were far more effective given her liver metastasis.

Thankfully, Linda responded very well to the treatment. Pains in her lower back and ribs improved significantly and her appetite improved. A CT scan showed a decrease in the size of her liver metastasis as well.

After two additional treatment cycles, scans revealed further improvement in the liver. A bone scan also revealed osteoblastic conversion of previous osteolytic lesions. This was an indication of new bone formation due to the slowing of cancer thanks to the chemotherapy.

Linda continued to feel better and did not require any pain medication. After a total of six cycles of chemotherapy, Linda's liver appeared normal on a CT scan. This was a pleasant and unexpected result for me, and a dream come true for Linda.

"Does this mean I am cured?" asked Linda at her office visit, with her husband seated beside her.

"You are in complete clinical remission," I explained, "which is an excellent sign."

"Can the cancer come back?" she inquired.

"Yes, it can come back... but I can't predict when or even if it will. A complete cure is not a realistic expectation; it's best to look at your cancer as a chronic condition. Your cancer has positive estrogen receptors, which means that it is feeding on your own hormones. We will start you on Tamoxifen to keep any microscopic cancer cells in check."

I put her on Tamoxifen as a maintenance treatment. When she reached menopause, I switched her to Anastrazole. She remained on that treatment for years and was still on it at the time of my retirement.

I followed up with Linda at regular intervals, reviewing her CT and bone scans until I retired in May of 2011. She was happy, active, and enjoying a good quality of life in remission at that time. She was very grateful that she had endured. Two of her friends had passed on from breast cancer and as she outlived each one, she realized again how lucky she has been. She continues to work full-time and hopes to retire by the age of sixty. She continues to take an annual family vacation to Kauai, Hawaii and has been able to see both of her sons graduate from college.

Linda kept in touch on a regular basis, even after I retired. When I told her about my own trip to Kauai in 2015 for my fortieth wedding anniversary, she sent me discs of several movies shot in Hawaii. In a recent email from Linda, received in late 2020, she informed me that she was still working full time and maintaining as normal a life as possible, given the limitations imposed upon all of us by COVID-19.

Is Linda cured? Probably not. To me, she perfectly exemplifies my assertion that a cure is not the only definition of hope. The message I gave Linda and her husband that first day we met is a message I have passed along to many patients with treatable cancers: hope for you is the improvement of both your quality and quantity of life.

The following is the letter I received when I first asked Linda's permission to include her story in my book:

> Oh, my goodness, I would be honored to be mentioned in your writing! It would make my family very proud also.
> I know that I have had an unusual journey with this disease. Many are not as lucky as I have been. I know it and so does my family. We feel very fortunate to still be able to share memories...
> I have been helped, supported and encouraged by others along the way. If I can be a source of encouragement for someone, that would make me very happy.
> Thanks! Linda.

Later, I received a couple of follow-up emails from Linda in response to a message I sent asking her how she and her husband were doing. The following is an excerpt:

> Your timing is always priceless! You are my angel on earth, sent to watch over me. We are good... I am on Faslodex and Piqray and things are holding steady for six months now. That is the longest that I've gotten from any single treatment since my recurrence in August of 2017...

The last I heard, Linda was still enjoying a good quality of life, including being able to spend time outdoors and working in her gardens.

Cancer As A Chronic Disease

Linda was one of many patients I had the privilege of treating who went on to enjoy quality of life in years well beyond their initial prognosis. A scenario like Linda's is not unique to breast cancer with metastasis.

Over the years, a growing number of cancers have begun to fall into the group seen as treatable. With newer targeted treatments, non-small-cell lung cancer patients and patients with melanoma can be long-term survivors as well. Prostate cancer patients, even those with bone metastasis, can survive for years now with proper treatment.

Other cancer types with long-term survival include those which can be completely cured with surgery such as cancers of the ovary and lymph glands, as well as chronic leukemias and some lymphomas. Cancer has, in many cases, become a chronic illness, which is manageable and treatable rather than being the death sentence it once was.

Strange as it may sound, the cure rates for cancer are actually higher than for almost any other chronic diseases. There is no cure for diabetes, chronic kidney failure, certain cardiac conditions, chronic arthritis, and other similar ailments. With newer and more targeted treatments, an increasing number of cancers are being converted into this category of chronic conditions.

Janice: Watching and Waiting

As previously stated, not all cancer diagnoses lead to death. Also, despite all the newly available targeted cancer treatments, there are still cases where treatment is not necessarily the best course of action for a patient with a diagnosis of proven malignancy. During my many years of practice, it was always a challenge to try to explain to patients why treatment was not a better option for them than to watch and wait.

I recommended the watch and wait course of action to Janice, a forty seven-year-old female patient who presented in 2005 with a white blood count of 38,000 (the reference range for normal is 4,000 to 10,000). Her hemoglobin and platelet counts were normal.

Further tests confirmed a diagnosis of chronic lymphocytic leukemia (CLL), the most common type of leukemia. CLL is also the most indolent type of leukemia with a relatively benign course for the majority of patients. There is no clinical evidence of benefit in treating the high white blood count in the absence of other symptoms. I witnessed some impressive longevity in patients with this diagnosis, two surviving for over twenty years.

Janice had no symptoms other than fear and anxiety, obviously understandable reactions to hearing the "C-word". An explanation backed up by literature which showed no benefit from treatment at this stage helped ease at least some of her anxiety. I followed up with periodic blood tests until my retirement in 2011 and found no need to subject Janice to treatment.

Her husband contacted me in July of 2019, fourteen years after Janice's initial diagnosis, to let me know that her white blood cell count was still elevated but stable. At that point, she was doing just fine and maintaining an active lifestyle without any need for treatment at all since her diagnosis. Although not very common, there can even be spontaneous remission observed in patients with this subset of leukemia.

The following is a letter I later received from Janice and her husband:

> *I really don't know how to tell you how grateful we are to you. We were both so frightened. Your calm and reassuring presence was a gift. I would be lying if I said I don't worry with my diagnosis. But knowing you are there to look at my labs and take care of me if necessary is so helpful. I feel totally confident putting myself in God's and your hands. Thank you.*

Jane: A Patient's Right to Choose

In June of 2000, Jane first came to me for a consultation. She was a twenty one-year-old college student who had noticed a lump in her neck three or four months before seeing me. After taking antibiotics for a week with no response, Jane was referred by her family doctor for a biopsy of the neck mass.

The mass turned out to be Nodular Sclerosing Hodgkin Lymphoma (NSHL) which is the most common and curable subtype of Hodgkin Lymphoma. This type of Hodgkin Lymphoma often has a genetic component, although Jane denied having any family history of the disease.

Jane was outwardly calm and answered all my questions without anger or frustration.

She admitted to having noticed more sweating, particularly in the evenings for the previous six weeks. This was a significant symptom, indicating aggressive behavior of her cancer.

She said she had not noticed any fever in herself but could not be certain, having not actually measured her temperature in that period. She reported having a good appetite but had lost ten pounds since she started noticing the night sweats just six weeks earlier.

A physical examination revealed several swollen although not tender marble-sized lymph glands on both sides of the neck and both axillae (armpits). I found no other abnormal lymph-node enlargement, and no enlargement of her spleen.

CT scans revealed enlarged lymph nodes in Jane's mediastinum, located between her lungs. CT scans of her abdomen and pelvis did not reveal any swollen lymph glands under her diaphragm. All blood tests were normal including the LDH and B-2 microglobulin markers for tumor activity.

Jane's cancer was staged as 2B, based on the presence of two or more groups of lymph nodes enlarged on the same side of the diaphragm, sweating in the evenings, and significant unintentional weight loss.

She was very clear and upfront with me from the very beginning, even before we had begun discussing treatment options. She said definitively, "I don't want chemotherapy!" This was significant since the standard treatment, then as now, for Stage 2B Hodgkin Lymphoma is chemotherapy combined with radiation for the involved field of swollen nodes.

The National Cancer Institute, a division of the Institutes of Health (NIH), estimates that there will be 8,830 new cases of Hodgkin Lymphoma in the United States in 2021, making up about 0.4% of all cancer cases nationwide[20]. With treatment that combines chemotherapy and involved field radiation, the five-year survival rate for stage 2B is extremely high with around a 75% chance for a complete cure.

Jane was adamant about limiting her treatment to radiation therapy, even knowing the high cure rate if it was combined with chemotherapy. Jane's mother felt helpless to change her daughter's mind. No amount of discussion with her mother or myself could sway Jane's mind, firmly made up against chemotherapy.

So, per her wishes, Jane received radiation therapy alone. Upon clinical examination four weeks after completion of her radiation, Jane showed complete remission with the disappearance of all previously swollen lymph glands. Her evening sweats had improved, and her weight remained stable. A CT scan confirmed complete remission, with her swollen glands in the mediastinum all returning to normal size.

I followed up with Jane at periodic intervals with physical examination and blood tests. Her mother was present at every office visit but did let her daughter do all the talking. Everything was fine for nine months.

At the nine-month mark, Jane noticed the recurrence of excessive sweating in the evenings, this time accompanied by a low-grade fever. These symptoms were suggestive of a return of the "B" aspect of her disease, which indicates the aggressive component of Hodgkin Lymphoma.

My examination of Jane during her office visit in April 2001 revealed enlarged lymph glands in her neck, both axillae, and groin area. Her disease had now progressed from stage 2B to clinical stage 3B.

Once again, I offered her standard chemotherapy known as ABVD, a combination of four different agents with an excellent chance of a positive response. Again, Jane refused. She had already decided on Rife Therapy, an unproven alternative treatment, and was adamantly opposed to chemotherapy of any kind.

The disappointment on Jane's mother's face was evident. She clearly disapproved of her daughter's decision. Unfortunately, she was helpless to change Jane's mind and said, resignedly, "She's an adult. I can't tell her what to do."

Rife machines operate at an electromagnetic frequency which is thought to be similar to that of cancer cells. It is purported to have curative potential with no side effects, unlike chemotherapy, which can have a variety of unpleasant outcomes in addition to the possibility of success. No current scientific literature reports reliable evidence for the use of Rife machines as cancer therapy and the treatment is still not FDA approved.

I understood the desperation Jane felt and her determination to pursue alternative therapy. I have seen that same desperation in many cancer patients both before her and since. It would have been much easier for me to understand Jane's decision had she been significantly older with advanced cancer and no effective treatment options available. Jane, however, was a college student in her early twenties, with her whole adult life ahead of her and to have her refuse a proven effective treatment option was difficult for me.

The combination of chemotherapy and radiation I recommended was potentially lifesaving. Although there would be more negative side effects in the short term, it would greatly increase her chances of having a long term to even consider. I made multiple attempts to convince Jane to opt for conventional treatments with proven benefits. Ultimately, I failed to convince her, as did her parents. I knew the inevitable ending Jane faced, unless a miracle occurred.

Unfortunately, no miracle was forthcoming and Jane's disease progressed. She died just four months later. This was a tragic end for a bright young woman with an excellent chance of long-term survival given the treatment options available to her.

I have asked myself many times in the years since losing Jane what more I could have done to prevent her untimely death from potentially curable malignancy. Sadly, when a patient has made up their mind not to pursue the recommended treatment, there is nothing further their physician can do. As long as the patient is given all the information, options, and likely outcomes, it is ultimately their choice how to move forward in treating or neglecting their disease.

Fortunately for my own emotional state, being an oncologist had enough rewards and happier outcomes to balance out the tragic ones like Jane's.

Paula: Same Diagnosis, Different Outcome

In July of 2001, I received a call from a physician I knew. He requested that I see his twenty five-year-old daughter, Paula, who had swollen lymph glands in her neck. An examination revealed enlarged non-tender nodes in her neck and axillary, with the largest being the size of a walnut. Paula admitted to having noticed increased sweating in the evenings for about three weeks. She said that she had not lost any significant weight.

A biopsy of a cervical node the following day confirmed a diagnosis of NSHL, the same subtype of Hodgkin Lymphoma that had taken Jane's life. A laboratory evaluation revealed mild anemia, unsurprising in a woman her age given her recent menstrual cycle. The remainder of her lab results were normal, including LDH, a marker for tumor activity.

A CT scan of Paula's chest, abdomen and pelvis showed enlarged nodes in her mediastinum only. Based on her history and CT results, she was staged as 2B, just as Jane had been when she first came to see me.

I recommended the same combination of radiation and chemotherapy that I had for Jane and felt encouraged by Paula's positive attitude and her willingness to undergo the standard treatment.

Paula had radiation therapy to her neck, axillae, and mediastinum followed by three cycles of ABVD chemotherapy, which was the standard treatment at that time. After the first two cycles, it was clear that the treatment was working well.

After radiation and three cycles of chemo treatments, Paula's evening sweating disappeared and the lymph-node swelling in her neck abated. A follow-up CT scan two months later revealed the complete disappearance of previously enlarged lymph nodes. Paula was in complete clinical remission. After two years of relapse-free follow-up appointments with me, Paula moved to Indiana for her career and while maintaining her remission, continued regular follow-ups with an oncologist in Indiana.

She sent me the following note in 2008, which made my day:

> Dear Doctor V,
> I had my check-up with my local oncologist two weeks ago. He says I am doing fine and wants me to get a scan and blood test. I remember quite vividly when I was preparing to start chemotherapy, you told me, 'Be brave and eventually this will all seem like a bad dream.' I thought about it a lot last fall and winter. Some days it kept me going.
> Thank you for all your help. I couldn't have asked for a more reassuring and understanding doctor.
> Sincerely, Paula

Since Paula's father was a physician of my acquaintance in Kalamazoo, it was easy for him to keep me updated on his daughter's health while I was still practicing there. She was free of cancer recurrence a full nine years after the completion of her treatment, after which I lost track of her.

What different results for Paula and Jane, two young women with the same diagnosis based almost solely on their attitudes! Although nobody can say for sure if Jane would have survived had she agreed to the recommended course of treatment, her chances would have been very high.

Bill: The Power of Positive Thinking

Fifty seven-year-old Bill was literally shaking during his first visit to see me regarding a possible diagnosis of leukemia in 2001. No one wants to see an oncologist, of course, but some show it more than others. Anxiety related to the fear of a coming cancer diagnosis is practically universal, especially at first.

Bill's white blood cell count was high at 22,000 per microliter (the reference range for normal is 4,000 to 10,000) with 30% blasts, or immature cells. His platelet count was low at 20,000 (the reference range for normal is 150,000 to 400,000). Platelets help clot the blood and prevent bleeding, so too few platelets meant he would be prone to excessive bleeding even from minor wounds. He was also anemic with a hemoglobin level of 8.8 g/dl (the reference range for normal is 12.5 to 15).

All of these factors taken together strongly suggested that Bill had acute leukemia. A bone marrow biopsy could help to confirm the exact type of leukemia. This was important information as the recommended treatment can vary widely depending on the type of leukemia a patient has.

Examination of Bill's bone marrow confirmed a diagnosis of Acute Myelogenous Leukemia (AML). The principles of treatment for AML involve total cell kill, meaning getting rid of not only the rapidly dividing cancer cells, but normal, seemingly healthy cells as well. This can result in increased risk for bleeding, severe infections, and even death.

During the most vulnerable period of this treatment, the entirety of a patient's blood cells are suppressed by the chemotherapy, leaving them quite susceptible. After chemotherapy, supportive treatments are administered to prevent a drop in the white blood cell count. Transfusions of platelets and red blood cells are also part of this supportive treatment, along with antibiotics if and when the patient develops any infection.

According to the American Cancer Society[21] most patients under the age of 60 who are otherwise in good health respond to induction chemotherapy (also known as remission induction). In this case, responding to treatment does not mean a full cure. In fact, a small number of leukemia cells often remain and must be treated with further therapy, known as consolidation, in order to prevent recurrence of the cancer.

Bill was in complete remission for two years before he relapsed, at which point he was referred to the University of Michigan for a second opinion. The physicians there elected to perform a bone-marrow transplant. A perfect bone marrow donor matches six out of six human leukocyte antigens (HLAs) with the recipient. The closest that Bill found was his son, a five out of six match.

In 2003, Bill underwent a successful bone-marrow transplant. He followed up at regular intervals over the next few years without any indication of a recurrence. He maintained his strength and continued to enjoy his favorite activities such as travel and golf.

Bill has kept in touch with me on a periodic basis. My most recent conversation with him was in December of 2019. He continues to be in great spirits and attributes his cure to his lifelong habit of positive thinking.

I never would have guessed when I first met Bill in 2001 that a complete cure would be his definition of hope but two decades later, it has become his reality.

Sherry: A True Inspiration

While standing in line at the airport in Miami, Florida in 2000, a woman approached me. I recognized her face but had forgotten her name.

"Hello, Dr. Vemuri! I'm Sherry, your patient with leukemia..." She went on to introduce her husband and their two children at which point, my memories returned.

Sherry had come to see me five years earlier when she was just a senior in college. She had acute myelogenous leukemia (AML), the same disease as Bill. It can be challenging for oncologists to treat this disease, and hard on patients to undergo treatment since the remission therapy can be so harsh on their bodies.

Fortunately, Sherry also responded well to treatment. She was given chemotherapy with Daunorubicin and Cytosine Arabinoside. Repeat bone-marrow biopsies confirmed she was in complete remission. Due to her young age and the high possibility of recurrence, her own healthy bone marrow was stored for the possible future transplantation since it was known to be a perfect match. This was before stem-cell transplants, a more comfortable procedure, were introduced.

Sherry moved away from Kalamazoo after her treatment. We had no further contact until our chance encounter in the Miami airport when I found out that she never needed a bone-marrow transplant.

While many AML patients initially respond to the treatment, the majority of them do not survive in the long run. The ASCO reports that the five-year survival rate for patients over the age of twenty is 26%.[22] Sherry's relative youth was a likely factor in her positive outcome; patients under the age of twenty have a significantly higher survival rate.

Seeing Sherry contented, in good health, and possibly cured forever really recharged my battery of hope. I felt happy for the rest of the day, and I smile even today as I write about her. It was a very pleasant surprise to discover that she did not even need the expected bone-marrow transplant.

Cindy: An Unexpected Recurrence

When Cindy first came to me in 2002 for cancer of the ovary, she presented with ascites, a fluid-filled abdomen which is common in patients with ovarian cancer.

Surgery is the primary treatment option for most ovarian cancers, with two main goals: staging and debulking the tumor. Staging is a diagnostic step which defines the spread of the cancer and debulking is the process of removing as much of a tumor as possible. Even when complete removal of a tumor is not possible, debulking it gives a patient their best chance of responding well to chemotherapy, thus improving their overall prognosis.

Cindy responded well to both surgery and chemotherapy, evidenced by her CA-125 tumor marker returning to normal after having risen to three times the normal level at the time of her diagnosis. CA-125 levels can increase in other abdominal cancers as well as in noncancerous conditions such as uterine fibroids. While not always accurate, monitoring CA-125 at periodic intervals can predict recurrence before the disease becomes obvious.

Cindy continued to be free of recurrence until the spring of 2005. At that time, a blood test performed in anticipation of her visit showed an elevated CA-125 level, suggesting a possible recurrence of her cancer. She was not reporting any physical symptoms and when I examined her, I did not find the expected increase in her abdominal girth from fluid accumulation. Yet, the increased CA-125 level was all the information I needed to know that Cindy's cancer had returned.

I will never forget seeing Cindy's husband's expression change from a smile to a frown of disappointment. He had brought me a handmade golf putter, which he then pulled out from behind his back. The gift was meant to be a present in celebration of the good news they anticipated receiving during the visit. The next several minutes were awkward for all three of us.

Just as I had expected it would, Cindy's abdomen soon filled up with fluid again, making her quite uncomfortable and loath to move around much. Rather than requiring her to come into the office to see me, I made house calls in order to treat her, bringing with me catheter vacuum bottles to withdraw the fluid from her abdomen and relieve some of the pressure. That made her feel somewhat better.

Toward the end stages of Cindy's cancer recurrence, we discussed alternative treatments. The chances of second and third line chemotherapy treatments helping her at that point were slim and were likely to have brought side effects which would only increase her discomfort and decrease her quality of life.

Ultimately, Cindy and her husband made the difficult decision to forego further treatment. Sadly, Cindy eventually passed away. She was in her early sixties at the time. In honor of Cindy and her husband, I still use the handmade putter they gave me.

Kevin: Golf Saved My Life

I met Kevin through his brother, my next-door neighbor. Kevin was a sixty one-year-old cancer survivor with the same diagnosis I now have: non-small-cell lung cancer. One day, he told me about his initial diagnosis. He went for a job interview in November of 2011 and had to undergo a routine chest x-ray as part of the physical exam required for the position. The x-ray showed a nine centimeter mass in his lungs.

I was quite surprised to hear that Kevin had been able to live with such a large lung mass without experiencing any noticeable symptoms such as pneumonia, severe cough, or shortness of breath.

"The mass they found on the x-ray led the doctors to order a CT scan of my lungs," explained Kevin. "The CT scan confirmed my worst fears. Everything moved very fast after that."

I did not treat Kevin myself, as I met him after my retirement, but I offered emotional support and made myself available for any questions he had; providing something of an unofficial additional opinion. Kevin saw an oncologist who found swollen lymph nodes on the right side of his lower neck. He ordered a needle biopsy of the lung mass and an MRI scan of the brain, which appeared to be normal.

"The doctor told me that I had stage 3B lung cancer, probably caused by smoking two packs of cigarettes a day for over twenty years," said

Kevin. "He explained that I had no marker on my cancer cells for targeted treatment. Then my daughter went onto Google and looked up my chances for survival. What she found shocked me. The search results said that I had only a 20% chance of survival and a 6% chance of being completely cured! I couldn't believe it."

Kevin's oncologist recommended radiation therapy and chemotherapy together. He would undergo radiation daily for six weeks and chemotherapy every three weeks for six treatments (Cisplatin and Etoposide). The doctor also informed Kevin about the long list of possible side effects that he might experience from the treatments. After reviewing Kevin's scans, I confirmed that the treatment being prescribed by his oncologist was standard and the same thing I would have done. I also encouraged him to continue playing golf, if that made him feel good.

"I decided to use my love of golf as an outlet," said Kevin. "I didn't get to play as often as I would have liked, due to weather, but I played as often as I could during radiation and chemo."

Kevin managed to tolerate his treatments without major side effects and even maintained his weight. Three months after completion of his treatment, a PET scan showed marked improvement.

"I continued to play golf as often as I could," he said. "I figured I would keep playing for as long as I had the strength to carry my clubs."

In August of 2012, six months after completing chemotherapy, Kevin received some excellent news: his PET scan was completely normal. At the time of his cancer diagnosis, his prognosis suggested a life expectancy of only two years. A second opinion at a major cancer center was even more discouraging, telling Kevin that he had just ten months to live.

Since then, Kevin has continued to see his doctor annually and undergo regular scans, which continue to show normal results. Kevin is yet another example of the variability of cancer behavior and outcomes, not to mention the power of maintaining a life filled with positive thinking and enjoyable activities.

Several times over the past eight years, Kevin has told me, "Radha, Golf saved my life! I golfed cancer out of my body. I have never felt better. I continue with my passion, playing golf every day when I am not at work."

Barbara: A Feel-Good Story

When Barbara came to see me for the first time, her cancer was small and limited to the breast. After a lumpectomy and five years of Anastrazole (Arimidex), an estrogen blocker, she faced very slim chances of recurrence. At her request, I saw her once a year, more for her own peace of mind than out of medical necessity. She was now eighty-one years old and in otherwise good health.

At one of her routine follow-up visits, Barbara brought a companion with her. She introduced him to me, saying, "Dr. Vemuri, I would like you to meet my boyfriend, Howard."

They went on to excitedly share their story, proof that love can come to any of us at any age. Barbara and Howard had attended high school together in Michigan. Howard had an eye for Barbara in their school days, but as often happens to high school sweethearts, they went their own ways after graduation.

Howard moved to Florida and got married, and Barbara married as well. Despite having a happy marriage, Howard never forgot his first love; Barb, as he called her. Throughout the years, he had kept track of her life from a distance. Five years before I met him, Howard's wife passed away. A few years afterward, Barbara lost her husband.

Since Howard had kept up with Barbara from afar, he knew about the passing of her husband and how to reach her afterward. They reconnected and their story had a happy ending that felt like something right out of the movies.

"That's what we wanted to share with you today," explained Barbara. "We're together and in love!"

"After a gap of over sixty years, I finally get to be with the girl of my dreams," said Howard. "Better late than never!"

"He's the greatest guy," said Barbara. "He even washes the dishes and cleans the house!"

Barbara was full of praise for Howard. They reminded me of a young newlywed couple. I will never forget them and their passion for each other.

Penelope: Miraculous Melanoma

In my long career as an oncologist, I only had two patients who experienced spontaneous regression. The first patient was a young woman in her mid-twenties named Penelope.

I first saw Penelope within a year of moving to Kalamazoo and starting my practice. Examination showed that she had a melanoma lesion on her leg below the knee. The lesion was surrounded by multiple visible melanoma nodules, evidence of metastasis. A biopsy confirmed the diagnosis of melanoma.

I found a clinical research study that Penelope was eligible to enter. The study involved one group receiving a chemotherapy treatment called DTIC and the other group receiving a placebo. Penelope declined to participate in the study not due to fear of being placed in the placebo group but because she was concerned about taking the chemotherapy.

She left my office without treatment. There was nothing more I could do for her unless she changed her mind and decided that she wanted to pursue treatment. Two years passed with no word from her at all. Then she called the office, asking to make an appointment to see me. I was happy to see her again.

When Penelope came in for her appointment, I examined her and could find no evidence that there had ever been a melanoma on her leg. "Did you get Laetrile?" I asked her. In those days of the mid-1970s, Laetrile was a popular alternative cancer medication made from apricot pits. As it was not (and still is not) approved by the FDA, it was not uncommon for patients to travel to locations such as Mexico in pursuit of the unproven therapy.

"No, Doctor," she said.

"Did you receive any other type of treatment?"

"No, I didn't."

"You didn't take anything?"

"No . . . it improved all by itself!" she explained.

Apparently, Penelope was one of those rare examples of spontaneous regression, sometimes thought of as a miracle. It was hard to believe but true, the evidence was right in front of my eyes.

I followed her case for another year or so, during which time she continued to be completely free of melanoma. I asked her if she wanted to come in for a follow-up visit and she replied that she was fine and would call me if the cancer returned and she needed to come in and see me. That was the last I heard from her.

Spontaneous Regression: A rare and wonderful phenomenon

Although rare, a patient may experience spontaneous regression or remission of their cancer. This phenomenon seems miraculous but does actually happen. Spontaneous regression is a partial or complete disappearance of cancer without specific treatment. Over the past 100 years, there have been multiple recorded isolated cases of this occurrence.

The most common mechanism attributed to this phenomenon is immunity; specifically, the immune response of the cancer patient's body. The theory is that certain patients produce unique antibodies that boost their immune system's response to cancer.

An article published in the journal *Medical Hypotheses*[23] attributes spontaneous regression to the following contributory factors: apoptosis (the death of cells which occurs as a normal and controlled part of an organism's growth or development), tumor microenvironment (the environment surrounding a tumor, including blood vessels, immune cells, etc.), and DNA oncogenic suppression (tumor suppressor genes which slow down cell division, repair DNA mistakes, or tell cells when to die, etc.).

Almost any type of cancer can go into spontaneous regression. This phenomenon is more likely to happen, however, certain types of cancer such as melanoma, kidney cancer, neuroblastoma (mostly in children), lymphoma, leukemia, and choriocarcinoma (a cancer involving the placenta which is found only in pregnant women).

Richard: Disappearing Kidney Cancer

In the late 1990s, Richard first came to see me. He was fifty-eight at the time and had been referred to me for kidney cancer. He had been experiencing classic symptoms of the disease: night sweats, fever, and sudden weight loss. He had lost thirty to forty pounds over the course of only six months and was so weak when he came to see me that he arrived in a wheelchair.

Richard had been sent to me because his cancer had metastasized to both lungs. CT scans had revealed a mass on one of his kidneys. I put two and two together and identified the kidney mass as the primary source of the cancer which led to the lung metastases.

"Unfortunately," I explained to Richard, "the night sweats and fever you're experiencing are indicative of an aggressive tumor."

He expressed interest in having the cancerous kidney removed in the hopes that it might improve his situation. The problem was, after losing so much weight, he was in no shape for such a major surgery.

I started him on a course of hyperalimentation, administering high-protein, high-calorie nutrients intravenously. In this way, I hoped to build him up to the point where he was strong enough to undergo the arduous kidney removal surgery. Thanks to a visiting nurse, Richard was able to get this treatment in the comfort of his own home.

After about a month to six weeks of treatment, he had regained some of his weight. Now that he was stabilized and deemed strong enough to undergo surgery, he was brought in for a nephrectomy to remove his cancerous kidney.

I followed up with Richard by ordering periodic scans. Three months after his nephrectomy, a scan showed that his lung spots had begun to diminish. At the six-month mark, the lung spots were further improved to the point where 80 - 90% had disappeared. After about nine months, his chest CT was completely clear. All the spots were gone! His appetite also improved, allowing him to gain back his lost weight.

This was an incredible outcome for both the patient and for myself as his physician. I attributed Richard's recovery to the immune mechanism often thought to be associated with spontaneous regression. Tumor-specific antibodies produced by the patient's body may also contribute to this phenomenon.

Richard, of course, did receive some treatment. There is no question that removing the original cancerous kidney had a major impact on the improvement of his health including the eventual disappearance of the lung spots. However, as his lungs were never targeted for treatment, this is another example of spontaneous regression.

I followed Richard at regular intervals. He continued to feel great. Intermittent scans remained normal. He resumed his usual work and remained healthy for years. I saw him for a follow-up visit a year or so before my retirement, and he was still doing just fine. He ultimately died when he was nearly seventy years old of a cause totally unrelated to his cancer: an acute heart attack.

CHAPTER 12

After Treatment

Things Doctors and Patients Should Discuss

As a cancer patient nears the end of treatment, it is understandable for them to want to put cancer behind them and focus on other, more positive, aspects of life. It can be tempting to skip doctor's appointments and say goodbye to the entire medical team, who may serve as a reminder of the most difficult time in a patient's life. In fact, after finishing treatment, a cancer survivor often wants nothing more than to never be thought of as a patient again. For several reasons, it is imperative that a patient continues to show up for their appointments and be prepared for important discussions to take place. It is advisable to prepare a list of questions in advance.

The cancer survivor will need to know what to expect as they go forward. It is important that doctor and patient discuss topics such as:

- prognosis and likelihood of cancer recurrence;
- steps which can be taken to prevent or decrease the likelihood of recurrence;
- long-term physical and/or emotional effects of the cancer and its treatment;
- strategies for keeping anxiety at bay;

- support groups and other similar resources;
- a schedule for follow-up visits with a primary care doctor and oncologist;
- strategies for general health maintenance after cancer treatment; and
- ways to maintain overall life balance and keep hope alive.

Changes Cancer Survivors Might Experience

Cancer is such an impactful occurrence and affects every aspect of a patient's life. It is common for cancer survivors to undergo a shift in their physical and emotional well-being, as well as in their outlook and lifestyle. These changes will vary from person to person but some which are common among cancer survivors include:

- having a renewed appreciation for life;
- noticing (or initiating) changes in relationships, as some connections become closer and others become more distant;
- becoming more accepting of themselves or, conversely, having trouble adjusting to changes in their body;
- living free of anxiety and worry about their health or living in constant fear of a relapse; and

Observing changes in the types of activities one enjoys, which can include a newfound vigor for certain activities or a loss of interest in others.

Cancer survivors may find that their lives have changed in a myriad of ways, some for better, some for worse. What is inevitable is that people are never quite the same once cancer is in their rearview mirror.

Coping with Changes After Cancer

ASCO's *Cancer.Net* website[18] recommends certain strategies for coping with the challenges and changes faced by cancer patients even after treatment has ended. For addressing emotional concerns and worries, they recommend first recognizing and acknowledging the changes that brought them about, and being proactive in seeking and finding the support needed to address them.

Sometimes such support might come in the form of information. A lack of information about what to expect going forward can give rise to anxiety. It is important to keep in mind, however, the sometimes dubious nature of "information" that can be found online. It may take more than one Google search to determine the veracity of statistics.

Another way to find emotional aid is a support group. For some, this means a group of survivors of the same type of cancer, for others it can just be the ongoing support of family and friends, which is invaluable to any cancer survivor.

As I have stated before, it is common for loved ones to be at a loss as to how to best support the patient, now survivor, in their lives. The cancer survivor must do their part to keep the lines of communication open and guide their loved ones in providing the type of loving support they need. Friends and loved ones are an essential part of keeping hope alive even after the treatment is over, often at that point, the emotional healing is just beginning.

Those who are supporting and caring for cancer patients and survivors also need to make sure they get the support they need for themselves. Those who care for cancer patients, whether in an institutional or home setting, often experience many of the same emotions, concerns, and worries as patients and their families. Caregivers and their needs are often overlooked, which can lead to burnout and resentment.

CHAPTER 13

Death Hits Close to Home

Losing My Father

I TREATED COUNTLESS TERMINALLY ill patients throughout my career in oncology. I pride myself in treating every one of them with compassion and empathy as they faced their own mortality and impending demise. Then the time came when I had to make gut-wrenching and heartbreaking decisions about the care of my own parents.

Both my mother and father were eventually diagnosed with cancer. There was no difference in the way I approached their situations from a medical point of view; as I told patients' families, I had no double standard. However, the emotional experience of having cancer hit so close to home was completely different when I was, in some ways, sitting on both sides of the desk.

In 1996, I made an emergency trip to India to see my nearly eighty-year-old father. He had been admitted to the hospital with extreme fatigue and generalized bruising. Right after landing in Hyderabad, I dashed to the hospital where my father had been admitted.

Nannagaru was happy to see me but not necessarily surprised. I had spoken to him on the phone the week before from my home in Michigan. He greeted me with a weak smile. After brief formalities, he wanted to know the name of the disease that had made him so sick.

Before I had a chance to respond, his doctor walked into the hospital room.

I introduced myself as the patient's son, an oncologist who had just arrived from the United States. The doctor requested that I become part of my father's medical-care team and asked me to take a look at his peripheral blood smear. My review of the smear revealed a white blood count of 29,000 (the reference range for normal is 4,000 to 10,000). His platelet count was markedly decreased at 9,000 (the reference range for normal is 150,000 to 400,000). This extremely low platelet count was the reason for his bruising and intermittent nosebleeds.

The doctor had initially diagnosed my father with adult Acute Lymphoblastic Leukemia (ALL). After reviewing all of my father's slides, tests, and medical records, I corrected this diagnosis to one of Acute Myelogenous Leukemia (AML).

AML is a form of malignancy in which the patient's bone marrow makes too many myeloblasts or immature neutrophils. This interferes with the manufacture of red blood cells and platelets, which causes anemia, bleeding, and bruising. These leukemia cells also lose their ability to fight infections.

My father's hospital bed told a grim story. I saw scattered spots of blood on his sheets, caused by his bleeding bruises. All it would take in a situation like my father's was a tiny bump almost anywhere on his body to start those bruises bleeding again. It was truly heartbreaking to see my father in that condition.

Men over the age of seventy are particularly prone to AML. This is especially true if they have been exposed to high levels of radiation but can also happen without any demonstrable cause. A bone-marrow biopsy is routinely done to confirm the diagnosis and provide other important information, including any chromosome abnormalities which may be relevant to treatment.

The standard treatment for AML is combination chemotherapy. Unfortunately, this type of chemotherapy kills not only leukemia cells but normal cells as well. While young, otherwise healthy, patients may be able to withstand this sort of treatment, mortality rates are very high for those of my father's age and constitution. This is even with supportive care including antibiotics as well as red cell and platelet transfusions.

It is important to me that every patient be given the facts in simple language that is easy to understand. By involving the patient in decisions about their own treatment, they feel empowered. This feeling of empowerment can be all that gives hope to terminally ill patients and we, as physicians, should not have the authority to take away all hope.

I took a deep breath and explained the pros and cons of chemotherapy to my own father, just as I had done so many times to strangers throughout my professional career. "Nannagaru," I said, "I've reviewed your laboratory values. I am sorry to tell you that you have Acute Myelogenous Leukemia. Your platelet count is very low. This is what is causing you to bruise and bleed easily. Platelets help to clot the blood. With a platelet count of only 9,000, you cannot clot."

My father asked me many follow-up questions related to chemotherapy, and I gave him the facts. I explained, "Chemotherapy is the treatment of choice, but unfortunately, it will kill the good cells along with your cancer cells. Your blood cell counts will drop even further. At your age, you may not recover from infection and bleeding. Also, this hospital lacks the ability to transfuse platelets when needed. That's a definite need in AML chemotherapy. They also lack a dedicated team to care for patients like you, who become prone to infection after chemo, due to your lowered white cells."

My approach with my father, the man I most respected, was no different than it would have been with any patient facing tough treatment options. I have always prided myself in being candid and compassionate, regardless of whether I was speaking to a patient or a member of my own family.

AML in the elderly has only a 5% five-year survival rate even though outcomes have been improving steadily over the years for those up to 75, patients in my father's age group remain low.[24] These days, newer, gentler treatments are available for elderly patients with AML who cannot tolerate standard chemotherapy but these options were not around a quarter-century ago.

I spent about twenty minutes explaining the situation to my father.

My explanation prompted him to do some deep thinking. I could see from his expression that he had not been expecting such dire news. He spent a few quiet moments analyzing the pros and cons of chemotherapy treatment as I had laid them out for him.

After giving the situation his careful consideration, he said with a little smile, "Radha, I have had a good life. I don't want to go through chemotherapy with the suffering and side effects. I am at peace."

As much as I obviously wanted my father to live, I was relieved when he made the decision not to undergo chemotherapy treatment as I did not want to see him suffer for such a slim chance of success. I was hoping he would come to that conclusion but had to allow him to do it on his own. Had my father asked me for my recommendation purely on medical grounds, I would have been honest but suggesting that my father forgo treatment would have likely left me with feelings of guilt. When he came to the decision on his own, it lifted a great burden from my shoulders as I was able, with a clear conscience, to fully support his wishes.

I was happy to know that my siblings and I would not have to watch our father suffer from bleeding, serious infections, and other side effects caused by chemotherapy creating a lack of adequate white blood cells as well as the inevitable fatigue that he would feel from the anemia as his red blood cells were destroyed.

My wife and I were on vacation in Jamaica when I received a call letting me know that my father had passed away. He died on February 12th, 1996, just a few days after being discharged from the hospital and sent home. He was seventy-nine years old.

I was not surprised to hear this sad news. Having recently seen my father in the hospital, I expected the inevitable, having had many patients in the same situation. I knew, however, that it was going to be a real challenge to explain my father's demise to my mother and siblings who had not seen him in his final stages of illness and did not know how quickly these things could progress.

Despite having extensive professional experience dealing with death, it is a very different experience and much more difficult to console one's own family. I was wrong when I thought I was ready for anything. In actuality, I was not nearly as prepared as I expected my experience to have made me for such a task. I repeated to myself the words taught to me by my father: "Everyone who is born is destined to leave this world."

I knew what was facing me, in terms of family responsibilities related to my father's funeral. I did not want Karen to have to go through the trauma that I would endure. Additionally, there would be ceremonies in which she would be unable to take part, so I did not request that she accompany me to India.

Karen returned to Michigan and I took the next available flight home to India to see my mother and siblings. As the eldest son, I was given the first option of performing the final end-of-life rituals for my father. If I had been unable to go for any reason, my next eldest brother would have performed the rituals. Given that my father and I were so close, however, It was important for me to do it myself.

In Hinduism, the dead are not buried, but always cremated. According to ancient Hindu tradition, I was expected to start the cremation process myself with the help of a priest. Witnessing my father's body go up in flames was even more traumatic for me than his death.

When I pass on, I too will be cremated, but I have made arrangements for my body to be taken to a local funeral home where it will be cremated out of sight by professionals. I would never ask my own son to go through such a traumatic process given the availability of modern options.

Each day for twelve days, I performed all necessary end-of-life rituals for my father. These were ancient Hindu rituals that are still performed in the Brahmin (priestly) class today. At the end of the twelve days, I returned to my duties as an oncologist in Michigan, ready to care for other people's fathers since I could do no more for my own.

Looking back now, I realize that I was much more traumatized at the time of my father's passing than I was on the day of my own cancer diagnosis in 2018. I miss my father every day and I thank him frequently for guiding me throughout my life. I still keep in mind his life lessons as they relate to my own diagnosis and eventual mortality.

Losing My Mother

Life returned to its normal routine until early 2004 when my mother was diagnosed with a pelvic malignancy with bladder invasion. Surgery was not an option for my mother due to pelvic extension, meaning that the cancer had traveled outside the organ where it originated. It was thought that my mother's cancer originated in her uterus but this was never definitively confirmed.

She underwent external pelvic radiation therapy and one cycle of chemotherapy. After treatment, my mother experienced severe pelvic pain. It was unclear what was causing it but I suspect that the radiation may have induced cystitis, which is inflammation of the bladder wall.

Pain control, rather than eradication of her cancer, became the primary goal of my mother's treatment. I wish that her pain had been better managed during her last weeks of life. Unfortunately, it was very difficult to obtain a prescription for narcotics in India at that time, due to concerns about patients becoming addicted. Most physicians in the country lacked adequate training in the use of narcotics for pain control. I was encouraged to see, on my most recent visit to India in January of 2020, well-established hospice teams caring for patients with pain under the supervision of trained physicians.

Over the course of six months, I made three trips to India in order to attend to my mother's poorly controlled pain situation. I carried what pain medications I could to her from the United States but was able to transport only small quantities due to strict regulations in place to prevent narcotic abuse.

Had my mother been in America, I could have placed her in a palliative care facility, but they were not available in India at that time. Fortunately, India has made great strides in that department. These days, they are attracting medical-tourism patients from all over the world, thanks to their ability to offer a high quality of care at lower prices than many other countries.

On more than one occasion, my mother's pain was so severe that she expressed to me that she would rather leave this world than continue to suffer. This heart-breaking statement was similar to sentiments I had heard from many terminally ill patients over the years. My mother had always been the sort of person to suffer in silence. In fact, I do not recall her really complaining about anything before that, which made her statement all the more telling of the severity.

On September 18th, 2004, at the age of seventy-eight, my mother passed away. She was mercifully delivered from her terrible pain to the great relief of all of her loving children.

My brother handled the end-of-life rituals for our mother. However, my experience with the end stages of my mother's life was much more traumatic than with my father's due to the severe pain she suffered. It can be devastating to families to witness a loved one go through such terrible pain and suffering and the emotional effects can last a lifetime.

My siblings and I all try to emulate our mother, who had love and compassion for everyone. I never once heard her express an unkind word or criticism of another human being. We all try to carry her legacy of love and compassion into our own relationships. Not surprisingly, all of her remaining children are incredibly close, even today, despite our advancing age, differing opinions, and varied geographical locations.

Guilt and Regret

When a family watches their loved one die after suffering from cancer and/or its treatments, they can be left with powerful feelings of guilt and regret. Surviving family members often feel that perhaps there was something more they could have done to prolong or save their loved one's life. These emotions do not necessarily have any basis in fact but can be quite powerful nevertheless. It is also common for surviving family members to realize belatedly that there were things they should have said and done while their loved one was still alive. These feelings of regret over the fact that it is now too late can be quite troubling.

When I think of guilt and regret in surviving family members, the daughter of one patient in particular comes to mind. I met her while attending the funeral of her mother, a very pleasant woman who died from metastatic stomach cancer. She underwent surgery to remove part of her stomach but unfortunately, the cancer returned in her liver six months later. Stomach cancer can and will metastasize to both the liver and the lungs. As her cancer continued to worsen, we discussed the pros and cons of chemotherapy, which she decided to undergo.

The patient tolerated treatment well. Both she and her husband were thankful that she survived for two and a half years. While that may sound like a short time, it was longer than the usual life expectancy for stage IV stomach cancer with liver involvement. I enjoyed an excellent relationship with both the patient and her husband. So, when my patient passed away, I attended her funeral. I would always do my best to attend the funeral of a patient with whom I had a close relationship.

While I was there, the husband introduced me to their daughter from California. Not once during the years that I was treating her mother's illness had I met this woman since she had not come to visit her mother in all that time.

When the daughter was introduced to me, the first thing she said sounded like an accusation. "Could you have kept my mother alive?"

Her father, with whom I had developed a great rapport, apologized profusely for his daughter's inappropriate comment.

I explained, "Two and a half years of survival for stomach cancer with liver involvement is excellent . . . and unusual." The woman's father nodded in approval as I continued, saying, "It is very tragic to lose a loved one, and I totally understand how you feel. I am very sorry for the loss of your mother. I wish you strength as you grieve." I understood that the daughter was dealing with feelings of guilt over failing to visit her mother during the last months of her life. I also knew that it was easier for her to put the blame on me, the doctor, for failing to keep her mother alive indefinitely, rather than focus on her own inaction and failure to show up during her mother's illness.

I came to think of the guilt and regret experienced by surviving family members as "daughter from California syndrome."

By contrast, I have received multiple positive letters from children of patients of mine who had passed:

> I would like to thank you so very, very much for the wonderful way you treated my father. I know you did everything humanly possible to stop the cancer. Unfortunately, this was really always out of our hands and in the hands of the one above.
>
> Your kindness and consideration helped to make Dad's last few days a little more bearable for him and the family. You are an inspiration to all those who work with and come in contact with you. I know through people's losses, you will be able to help others and put some smiles back on people's faces. That's what it's all about. Thanks again for everything.

~ * ~ * ~ * ~

> We all thank you for the wonderful care you gave to Mom during her illness and leading up to her death. We felt secure with the medical treatments you advised. Coupled with that was your sensitivity and perception to Mom's emotional needs, and the compassion and kindness you showed her.
>
> All through her life, she showed us courage, hope, patience, perseverance, a love for life, and caring for others. And she always seemed to be at peace with herself.
>
> Thank you for your last talk with her that morning at the hospital. During one of my last conversations with her at Rose Arbor, she said, "This is easier than I thought it would be." Thank you for making this true!

End of Life Concerns and Preparations

> *"For the soul, there is neither birth nor death."*
> ~ Bhagavad-Gita (Chapter Two)

I have heard various versions of the quote "In Europe, death is inevitable. In America, it is optional!" It has been attributed to Europeans and Americans, to philosophers and doctors. No matter who said it originally, however, the sentiment remains valid.

As an oncologist, I have seen more deaths than most people. In my experience dealing with elderly patients, especially those in their eighties and nineties, I often encountered that "death is optional" perspective.

The truth is that everyone born is destined to someday leave this world. This is a fact of life that many healthy people manage to avoid facing. Those diagnosed with cancer, however, must face their own mortality and deal with end-of-life concerns and preparations. If they do not, these responsibilities can fall on the shoulders of their unprepared family members.

One patient of mine, William, was eighty-eight years old and had advanced lung cancer. After exhausting all treatment options, William's cancer continued to progress. Since he did not have a Living Will, it was left to his children to consider the available options and make decisions on their father's behalf.

William's son wanted to do everything he could to keep his father alive even a moment longer, including putting him on a ventilator. His daughter, on the other hand, did not want to go to extraordinary lengths to unnaturally extend her father's life; she did not want him to endure any more discomfort. This type of scenario where family members have opposing ideas related to an ailing relation's medical situation is all too common and can result in strained relations among family members.

For this reason, it is a good idea for all patients admitted to the hospital to have a Living Will. Living Wills and Advanced Directives are legal documents reflecting a patient's preferences for medical care in the event that they cannot make their own medical decisions. Unexpected end-of-life occurrences can happen at any age, so all adults really ought to prepare these documents.

CHAPTER 14

The End of An Era

Retirement

My retirement was not something I had planned long in advance. In 2007, Karen and I visited Greensboro, Georgia for a vacation. While we were there, I played golf at a local resort. We met members of the golf club who were friendly and we had a wonderful time. We returned the following year and very much enjoyed ourselves again. So, we bought a house there. At that point, we knew it would eventually be our home in retirement, as Karen was adamant about not maintaining two houses in the long term, but there was no particular date in mind for us to make the move.

In November of 2010, while I was recovering from knee replacement surgery, we came to our house in Greensboro for rest and rehabilitation. While there, I felt it was time to start paying more attention to my physical health and well-being. I also wanted to spend more time with Karen, who has been such an important, supportive, loving part of my life. It was at that time that I really made the decision to retire.

I officially retired in April of 2011 and we were fortunate enough to find a buyer for our house in Kalamazoo even before officially putting it on the market. We decamped to Georgia within a month.

The summers in Georgia were very hot and I had become unaccustomed to the weather, having spent the last forty years in

Michigan. So, in 2012, I decided to accept a two-month job as a locum tenens in Petoskey, Michigan, filling in for an oncologist there who was on leave. Karen came with me to Michigan to escape the worst of the Georgia summer heat. The summer weather in northern Michigan was perfect. It stayed light outside until nearly 10:00 p.m., which allowed me to play golf in the evenings after I left the hospital. I very much enjoyed working there for the summer. I became quite fond of the staff and made some new friends. I had a truly great time, both with patients and the activities I was able to pursue. It was a good opportunity to help ease me into being fully retired.

Karen and I are very much enjoying our life here in Greensboro. We live surrounded by nature in a peaceful environment where I can enjoy golfing and other outdoor activities that contribute to my life balance and overall well-being. Occasionally, I will get a call from someone seeking my medical opinion and I always appreciate those opportunities to use my knowledge and experience to help others.

During my career treating cancer patients, I experienced tremendous satisfaction. I very much enjoyed interacting with my patients, and felt I was fulfilling my dharma, the Hindu concept of my sacred duty and one of the main aims in life. I periodically received welcome surprises in the mail, like the following, which confirmed for me that the path I took whether it was chosen for me or by me, turned out to be the perfect option.

> We would like to thank you for your years of dedicated service to the cancer community. We believe it is because of your expertise and caring that our family has been able to enjoy so many years with our parents and grandparents.
>
> You have been a part of our lives since 1987 and we will forever be grateful for the kind, caring and professional way in which you treated our mother and father. Enjoy your retirement! You have definitely earned it and you will definitely be missed.

The End of An Era

~ * ~ * ~ * ~

I think of you often. It is such a privilege to have you for my friend! I am so glad you are helping patients to understand about their conditions and educate the public about cancer. You have wonderful insight into what people need in order to be able to deal in a positive way with their condition.

I must tell you, you definitely have made life better for others. You really make a great difference! Thank you for being you.

~ * ~ * ~ * ~

When Gary and I first received the diagnosis of my cancer, there was never any question of who we wanted to treat me. After experiencing the tender care that you had given to both of Gary's parents over the past decade, we knew you were the only person we wanted to help us get through this challenge.

Let me explain. To begin with, you never see your patients as throat cancer or lymphoma or colon cancer. Rather, you see each patient as an individual who happens to be ill. You treat the whole person, not just the disease.

This was clearly evident whenever we hit a bump in the road which prolonged my treatment. I didn't have to tell you how badly I wanted to be home. You always knew. In fact, your empathy made the delays much easier to bear. Your ability to treat us as an individual *family has made us feel like you are, indeed, a member of our family.*

Next, like any good educator, you always had time for us. You never made us feel rushed during an appointment, even though we always seemed to have a bazillion questions! Your ability to synthesize information and easily explain the options are the hallmark of an excellent teacher.

How lucky we were to have both a doctor and an educator—someone who has helped take the fear and mystery out of cancer. Your ability to guide us through the maze was extraordinary.

Also, your years of experience were always very comforting. There isn't much you haven't seen, given the thousands of patients you've treated over the years. You had an innate ability to predict when I was about to crash. Your knowledge of how to avert potential problems only reinforced the idea that I was in the hands of an expert.

I will be forever grateful to have been under your care. Thank you for saving my life.

Listening To and Caring For Patients

Although I have been retired for many years now, I do my best to keep up with medical journals in my field. It is a way to keep my mind active in the same way that golf and tennis keep my body in good shape.

I know that I am far from the only physician who knows the importance of maintaining core principles for both the physical treatment and emotional well-being of patients. An article in the ASCO Post[25] recently caught my eye. because it listed some of the very principles to which I always adhered while practicing medicine, including:

- promoting a model for enhanced listening to and caring for patients;
- developing a new science to better operationalize and communicate clinical uncertainties; and
- rethinking symptoms and recognizing that many are unexplained, self-limited, and can benefit more from careful approaches than indiscriminate testing, among others.

These principles resonate with me both as a physician and as a patient. We must always remember that every patient is an individual. We cannot assume that his or her cancer will follow a typical path. We must support patients, and most importantly, we must listen to them about their goals.

In the following letter, a patient of mine comments on how much it meant to her to be listened to and treated like an individual. I believe the importance of this cannot be overstated.

> Let me begin by saying thank you. At a time in my life when I had a storm raging within me, based on a foundation of fear, you were the person who brought calm to that storm. Over the past ten years, you have given excellent medical care. Not once did I doubt that I had the right oncologist on my team.
>
> You taught me a lot about the relationship between a doctor and a patient. You always listened to each and every word I had to say. You expressed to me that I have to be in charge of my decisions, and you taught me that it was not for a doctor to decide these things for me.
>
> Thank you. I commend the manner with which you always approached me. Kindness, concern, knowledge and truth were the elements you brought into that room. You always had a smile or a gentle touch on the shoulder. When

you shook my hand, you would hold that touch for just a tiny moment longer than others. I felt calmer when you did that.

In today's world, not enough people actually take the time to connect on the human level. Thank you! You gave me encouragement and hope. I still wake up with that hope every day.

I was at a funeral recently where I heard a pastor speak some words that touched me more than any I had heard in church before. I, like so many [cancer] survivors have always asked the question, Why me?

My question was answered with the words I heard: 'When we have many struggles in our life, we gain endurance from those struggles. Through that endurance, we build character. It is from that character, that we are then able to find hope.'

Hope: the one thing that every cancer survivor needs and must be able to find!

Afterword

It has been years now since my diagnosis of lung cancer with brain metastasis, and I am still alive and reasonably well. I am aware that I am not out of the woods yet, even though I am very functional. My end will come someday, but hopefully not soon.

For a while, I was dealing with symptoms related to the effects of the targeted radiation to my brain. The most noticeable effect was on my sense of balance although fortunately, this has improved greatly in the last year. When it was happening, it was a huge adjustment for me as I have always been reasonably agile and am unused to such things preventing me from activities I enjoy such as playing tennis. Of course I missed that game greatly and am fortunately back at it now but it was not the only activity affected; my balance even faltered during everyday activities such as walking. When walking quickly, particularly downhill, I could lose my balance and fall forward. This happened two or three times in a single month. Anyone can stumble, of course, regardless of their health, but both the frequency and novelty of this problem was of concern to me while it was going on last year.

One of these falls took place on a golf course as I was walking downhill. The grass was slippery from being wet and after falling down, I had a particularly hard time getting up, due to both the terrain and my balance issues. A couple walking by helped me up and generously drove me home. People like them remind me that there are wonderful people in the world and that I ought to focus on the good in life. Keeping a positive outlook is very important to me.

Generally speaking, my symptoms are minor. Every day, I walk three or four miles without even leaving my own home, just by moving around my living room and small home gym. Sometimes I run back and forth across the basement. I also do jumping jacks. I test myself as I am walking, asking myself whether my steps are identical in length. I walk around in circles so much that Karen sometimes asks me, "Are you getting dizzy yet?"

In January of 2020, I was given stereotactic radiosurgery (SRS) to a tumor in the right frontal lobe of my brain. This led to me developing necrosis, or scar tissue. Though the MRI of my brain continues to suggest that the scar tissue itself might be the cause of those symptoms, residual cancer cannot be completely ruled out.

A radiation specialist recommended brain surgery to confirm or rule out residual cancer in the area of necrosis. He also recommended treatment with Gamma Optune therapy. My medical oncologist, on the other hand, felt that such a surgery could have adverse effects on my brain function because the treatment had the potential to injure parts of my brain that are, at this point, functioning normally. He also felt it could potentially exacerbate both my issues of balance and cognition. Really, the latter are remarkably minor, given my medical condition and I saw no reason to tempt fate in such a way.

My oncologist recommended I.V. treatment with Bevacizumab (Avastin) a VEGF (vascular, endothelial growth-factor inhibitor) which has been shown to help with necrosis. The hope is that it will inhibit further growth of both the scar tissue and any possible tumors. Avastin is not a new medication. In fact, I was already quite familiar with it. During my years in practice, I regularly prescribed it for patients with metastatic cancers, including lung cancer like my own. I was not aware, however, of the medication's benefit for radiation necrosis. My oncologist supplied me with an article on the topic, and after reviewing it, I determined that I concurred with my oncologist's treatment plan. Maintaining a good quality of life is far more important to me than prolonging my life by a few months while experiencing possibly debilitating side effects from more toxic chemotherapy. I am thankful to my oncologist for discouraging me from having brain surgery.

The Avastin is being given as an I.V. injection every two weeks at my oncologist's office. I have already received the first of four infusions. I hope (and expect) to finish the treatment without any serious complications. I am encouraged by the fact that I have had no significant negative reaction so far. I have developed mild to moderate high blood pressure, which is a known complication and treatable with a common medication. After the treatment concludes, we can determine how my brain has responded to it.

I am thankful to my oncologist for both his knowledge and his interest in my care. As he promised at our initial visit, he is treating me like his own family.

Given the lack of major symptoms, I am experiencing very little sadness and very little fear about my mortality. As long as I am getting the best treatment, which I genuinely believe I am, I know that I am able to accept any outcome.

At times I have asked myself, do my friends and family think I am in denial over my terminal illness? Is that how they interpret it when I do not share sadness or fears about my mortality with them?

I know that I cannot control what they think of course, only how I think and act and I can only hope that they know me well enough to attribute my lack of negative emotions not to denial but rather to my lifelong practice of detachment without indifference, which I learned in my early life. It is responsible for my ability to maintain a good quality of life despite having stage four metastatic cancer. I also attribute this good quality of life to my maintenance of a healthy daily routine.

Both scientific research and my personal experience tell me that the practice of regular exercise is highly beneficial. I have noticed benefits that are physical, psychological, emotional, and cognitive in nature. I believe that the key is to set achievable goals in exercise as in other facets of life.

I am not particularly concerned about death; I certainly hope it does not come any time soon, of course, but I know that it is an inevitability and have fully accepted that. I am, however, concerned about suffering and becoming a burden on Karen and the rest of my family if I lose brain function as I decline. That would be very traumatic, especially for my wife. I do not dwell on such negative outcomes, as it does no good for anybody. I remain positive and hopeful that the infusion treatment I am currently receiving will help the necrosis and improve my residual neurological symptoms. As for pulmonary symptoms, I have not had any, despite the source of my cancer being in my lungs. In fact, thanks to regular use of a pulse oximeter, I can confidently say that my blood oxygen level has not fallen below 95% (the general cutoff for a normal reading).

Every life has its challenges. That is the nature of living. Currently, we are all suffering the devastating toll of the COVID-19 pandemic. The restrictions due to this pandemic have prevented me and my wife from spending time with our grandchildren who live across the country in California. We miss them very much.

I have a brain MRI and whole body CT scan scheduled for later this month, the findings of which will determine if I can continue to be so active or if I need to start preparing myself for the final stages of my life. Whatever the outcome, I am at peace. I continue to focus on positive thinking and hope. These are the not-so-secret keys to having total peace of mind. Fortunately, I have plenty of both. I have had a good life and I hope to continue to have a good quality of life for as long as possible

Never lose hope! It is a powerful prescription; not only for those who are ill but for everyone.

About the Author

RADHAKRISHNA (RADHA) VEMURI, M.D. was a practicing oncologist for thirty-five years. While practicing, Dr. Vemuri treated all his patients with compassion, involved them in all discussions related to their treatment and care, and did his best to offer hope to every single patient, regardless of the stage of their disease.

The author was raised in Hyderabad, India as one of eight children. His family is of the Brahmin (priestly) class. His father, forbidden to pursue his own dream of being a doctor due to traditional caste restrictions, encouraged his eldest son to do so in his stead.

Dr. Vemuri attended the Institute of Medical Sciences Osmania Medical College in Hyderabad, India from 1964 to 1970 and graduated at the top of his class. After completing a compulsory internship in India in 1971, Radha immigrated to the United States in July of that same year. Upon arriving in the United States, he did a second internship from 1971 to 1972 at Highland Park Hospital in Detroit, Michigan. From 1972 to 1974, he was an internal medicine resident at Detroit's Sinai Hospital.

From 1974 to 1976, Dr. Vemuri did his fellowship in oncology at Henry Ford Hospital. In 1975, he married Karen Machemer. In 1976, they moved to Kalamazoo, Michigan where they resided until his retirement in 2011.

From 1976 through 2011, Dr. Vemuri held the position of Clinical Professor of Medicine, College of Human Medicine, Michigan State University. He received the Michigan State University (MSU) Teacher of the Year award multiple times; voted for by residents in training. In

1988, he also received MSU's Community Teacher of the Year award. In 1997, Dr. Vemuri was awarded the American Cancer Society's Community Service Award.

In 1994, Dr. Vemuri became the founding medical director of the West Michigan Cancer Center, a position he held until his retirement. He considers himself fortunate to have had such a dedicated and wonderful staff at the West Michigan Cancer Center, all of whom devoted themselves to creating an environment that addressed all aspects of the patients' well-being, especially their need for hope.

In 2018, the cancer doctor became a cancer patient himself. He notes that he has not slowed down despite having stage IV non-small cell lung cancer. He continues to offer medical consultations to friends and family in retirement and maintains an active lifestyle by walking, playing golf and tennis, and exercising both at home and at the local gym. His life remains as fulfilling as it was during his career.

Acknowledgments

First and foremost, I want to acknowledge my beloved wife, Karen... I cannot thank you enough for our forty-six years of marriage together. In my early years of oncology practice, you recognized the stress involved in caring for sick and dying patients and encouraged me to play sports as a way of maintaining balance in my life. You continue to be a source of great encouragement to me during my own cancer treatments. I am deeply grateful.

To my dear daughter, Neena Kalyani... Thank you for your help throughout this book; with ideas during the early stages, with editorial and technical help from the initial writing phase through to the final draft, for knowing how to put my thoughts into words and understanding what I mean even when nobody else does. Thank you for educating me about document formatting and making it easier for me to organize chapters, and for all your help with my gadgets. You are always my special daughter and this book would not have been possible without you.

To my dear son, Naveen Krishna... Thank you for your comments and support throughout the writing process and in the years before. Thank you for the thoughtful foreword which makes me proud to be your father. You have given me enormous satisfaction and more happiness than you will ever know. I'll never forget the fun we've had traveling as a family and playing tennis tournaments as partners. You have always played a key part in the balance in my life. I will always remember and cherish the memories we made and the photos of us as champions.

To my brother Ramesh . . . Thank you for introducing me to Google Docs and helping me understand how to put my thoughts into words and properly construct sentences to do so. I appreciate your support, input, and feedback throughout the process of writing this book.

To the rest of my dear family . . . Thank you all for your continued love and support, not only while I was writing this book but throughout my life, especially during my recovery periods. You will always be loved.

To my medical school buddies . . . Thank you for your friendship and brotherhood since 1964. Thank you also for visiting me to check on my health during my initial treatment and for continuing to check on me in our regular Zoom calls.

To my tennis and golf friends . . . I cannot thank you enough for your support and your prayers for my health.

To Carla, administrative assistant at WMCC . . . You were very helpful to me during my tenure at the Center, and you continue to help by providing some of the pictures I've included in this book. Thank you.

To my patients who allowed me to use their stories . . . Thank you for being willing to share your stories as an inspiration to others.

To Jennifer Patton . . . Thank you for your efforts on the early draft of this book. I appreciate your help. And to Coach Patton, thank you for being such a good friend and a good person. My grandson Milo still reminds me of the fun he had riding a horse with you.

To writer Vivien Cooper . . . Thank you. This book project was at least twenty years in the planning stage. Its completion would not have been possible without your help and guidance during the writing process. Along the way, you became my dear friend.

Works Cited

1. Mahendran R, Chua SM, Lim HA, et al. "Biopsychosocial correlates of hope in Asian patients with cancer: a systematic review." *BMJ Open* 2016;
2. Corn, Benjamin et al. "The Science of Hope." *The Lancet Oncology*. September 2020
3. Reeve, Christopher. Nothing is Impossible: Reflections on a New Life. Random House. 24 September 2002
4. Groopman, Jerome E. Anatomy of Hope: How People Prevail in the Face of Illness. Random House. 1 January 2004
5. Brody, Howard. "Hope." *Journal of the American Medical Association (JAMA)*. 25 September 1981
6. Kubler-Ross, Elisabeth. On Death and Dying. Scribner. 2 July 1997
7. Vemuri, Radhakrishna and Cavallo, Jo. "Having Cancer Has Not Affected Me in Any Negative Way." *The American Society of Clinical Oncology (ASCO) Post*. 10 August 2020
8. 3 Life Lessons We Can Learn From the Bhagavad Gita. yogiapproved.com/om. Accessed 29 April 2021.
9. Radon | US EPA. epa.gov/radon. Accessed 30 June 2019
10. The Radon Information Center. radon.com. Accessed 30 June 2019
11. Moving Us Closer to Osler. closter.org. Accessed 2 May 2021
12. Phillips KA, Ospina NS. "Physicians Interrupting Patients." *Journal of the American Medical Association (JAMA)*. 4 July 2017

13. Coping and Living Well During Cancer Treatment. cancer.org/treatment/survivorship-during-and-after-treatment/coping.html. Accessed 25 September 2021

14. Medscape.com (login required).

15. Fry, Erika and Schulte, Fred. "Death by a Thousand Clicks: Where Electronic Health Records Went Wrong." *Fortune*. 19 April 2019

16. Gilligan, Adrienne M et al. "Death or Debt? National Estimates of Financial Toxicity in Persons with Newly-Diagnosed Cancer." *The American Journal of Medicine*. 12 June 2018

17. Cancer Diagnosis Puts People at Greater Risk for Bankruptcy. https://www.fredhutch.org/en/news/releases/2013/05/cancer-diagnosis-greater-risk-bankruptcy.html. Accessed 6 November 2021

18. Coping With Cancer. https://www.cancer.net/coping-with-cancer. Accessed 7 November 2021

19. Greisinger AJ, Lorimor RJ, Aday LA, Winn RJ, Baile WF. "Terminally ill cancer patients. Their most important concerns." *Cancer Pract*. 1997 May-Jun

20. Adult Hodgkin Lymphoma Treatment. https://www.cancer.gov/types/lymphoma/hp/adult-hodgkin-treatment-pdq. Accessed 23 November 2021

21. Typical Treatment of Adult Myeloid Leukemia. https://www.cancer.org/cancer/acute-myeloid-leukemia/treating/typical-treatment-of-aml.html. Accessed 23 November 2021

22. Leukemia - Acute Myeloid - AML: Statistics. https://www.cancer.net/cancer-types/leukemia-acute-myeloid-aml/statistics. Accessed 23 November 2021

23. S.A. Hoption Cann, J.P. van Netten, C. van Netten, D.W. Glover. "Spontaneous regression: a hidden treasure buried in time." *Medical Hypotheses*. Volume 58, Issue 2, February 2002

24. Thein, Mya S et al. "Outcome of older patients with acute myeloid leukemia: an analysis of SEER data over 3 decades." *Cancer* vol. 119,15 (2013)

25. Lim, Andrea J et al. "10 Patient-Centered Principles for More Conservative Cancer Diagnosis." *ASCO Post*. 10 March 2019